Unlocking Regeneration: The HypnoCell® Method for Neuroplastic Healing

Unlocking regeneration : The Hypnocell® method for neuroplastic healing
Copyright © 2025 by Dr. Lucy Coleman
Coleman Publishing
ISBN : 978-1-949545-37-1
Contact info : www.hypnocell.com
10 9 8 7 6 5 4 3 2 1

Unlocking Regeneration: The HypnoCell® Method for Neuroplastic Healing

A clinical guide to hypnosis, brain plasticity, and the science of cellular renewal

Dr. Lucy Coleman

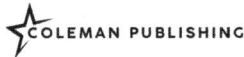

COLEMAN PUBLISHING

"When the mind believes in regeneration, the body remembers how."

The mind doesn't just witness the body—it instructs it. Every thought and emotion sends signals that shape cells, guide healing, and write tomorrow's biology. Change your mind's story, and you begin to change everything.

□

Important note on the use of hypnosis techniques and the term "healing"

The techniques described in this book have been used by patients who have reported significant improvements in their physical, emotional, or mental well-being. However, it is essential to understand that individual responses to therapeutic practices vary greatly, and outcomes cannot be guaranteed.

I strongly recommend that any practice involving hypnosis, neuroplasticity, or guided meditation be conducted under the supervision of a qualified professional, especially when pre-existing medical, psychiatric, or chronic conditions are present.

Throughout this book, the term *"healing"* is used to describe a state of noticeable improvement or perceived well-being experienced by the patient. This term is not intended to imply a cure in the conventional medical sense, nor should it be interpreted as a substitute for any medical, pharmacological, or psychological treatment prescribed by healthcare professionals.

Therapeutic hypnosis and neuroplasticity tools may produce subjective experiences of health or emotional relief, such as reduced stress, pain management, and enhanced emotional regulation. These effects, while potentially powerful, do not guarantee the full resolution of any diagnosed medical condition.

This book is intended to educate, empower, and support, not to diagnose or treat medical disorders. Any decisions regarding starting, changing, or stopping a medical treatment should always be made in consultation with your healthcare provider.

Contents

·····●·●·●·····

Introduction

A new paradigm in healing

For decades, modern medicine has operated within a reductionist framework—dividing the body into organ systems, categorizing diseases by symptoms, and treating those symptoms as isolated malfunctions to be corrected. This model excels in acute care: when an artery is blocked, it must be cleared; when an infection is raging, antibiotics can save a life. But this same approach begins to falter in the face of chronic, complex, or recurrent conditions.

Illnesses like autoimmune disease, metabolic dysfunction, infertility, chronic fatigue, fibromyalgia, depression, and neurodegenerative disorders often resist linear diagnosis and pharmacological fixes. In these cases, patients are too often shuffled between specialists, their labs "within normal limits," yet they feel far from well. Eventually, they hear phrases like:

"We can't find anything wrong."

"Your symptoms are probably stress-related."

"Let's try another medication."

Or worse, "It's all in your head."

But what if it actually is in the head—not as imagined illness, but as disrupted communication between the brain and the body?

Symptoms as bio-intelligent signals

The truth is: your body is not failing—it's speaking.

Symptoms such as chronic pain, anxiety, insomnia, hormonal irregularities, infertility, and digestive upset are not mere mechanical errors. They are informational signals, often originating from unresolved stress, emotional imprints, environmental triggers, or outdated neural patterns.

These signals get encoded into the nervous system and—if left unaddressed—become habitual neural loops. The longer the loop persists, the more it shapes biology. Over time, that loop is reinforced not just emotionally, but structurally: through synaptic wiring, altered immune activity, and gene expression.

Yet most conventional treatments aim to suppress these signals rather than decode them.

We've been asking, "How do we stop this symptom?" when we should be asking, "What is the body trying to say—and what does it need to return to coherence?"

Toward a more intelligent medicine

This book invites you to shift from a passive model of care—where healing is outsourced—to an interactive paradigm, where healing emerges from within, activated by insight, intention, and the right tools.

This new model recognizes that:

The body is plastic, not fixed.

The brain is capable of rewiring itself.

Cells respond not only to chemicals, but to frequencies, emotions, and beliefs.

Healing is not linear—it is adaptive and multidimensional.

The HypnoCell® Method is based on this understanding. It merges clinical hypnosis with the principles of neuroplasticity, emotional integration, and regenerative biology. It sees symptoms not as flaws to silence but as codes to be understood and updated.

In the chapters that follow, you will learn to see your mind not just as a thinking machine, but as a tool for biological reprogramming. You will learn how to engage with your symptoms—not fearfully, but curiously—and how to direct your nervous system back into safety, balance, and regeneration.

This is not wishful thinking or mystical ideology. This is science, evolving beyond the mechanical model, and stepping into the era of informational healing.

Let's rewire not only the brain—but how we think about healing itself.

The emerging science of mind–body medicine

For centuries, healing traditions from various cultures—Ayurveda, Traditional Chinese Medicine, Indigenous rituals—have emphasized a holistic view of health, one in which the body, mind, and emotions are deeply intertwined. Only recently has Western science begun to catch up, thanks to breakthroughs in neuroscience, epigenetics, and psychoneuroimmunology.

These fields converge on a critical realization:

The mind is not just a bystander in health—it's an active participant in cellular behavior.

Modern imaging technologies, like fMRI and PET scans, allow us to witness in real time how thoughts, beliefs, and emotions trigger measurable changes in brain activity, hormonal output, and immune modulation. The implications are vast: healing cannot be limited to pharmacology or surgery—it must also consider how the brain processes experience and meaning.

What the research shows

Hypnosis modulates neural connectivity in real timeClinical studies using brain imaging demonstrate that during hypnotic states, connectivity shifts between key networks—particularly the default mode network, salience network, and executive control system. These changes correlate with increased focus, reduced pain perception, and enhanced neuroplasticity. Hypnosis, it turns out, is not sleep—it is a highly focused neurobiological state that primes the brain for change.

Belief, expectation, and guided imagery influence biological responses.

The placebo effect is no longer dismissed as psychological fluff. It's a validated mind-body mechanism that activates endorphins, modulates cytokine levels, and can accelerate healing. Guided imagery and suggestion amplify this process by shaping internal expectations and redirecting physiological pathways.

Brainwave entrainment induces neuroplastic remodeling.   Techniques like binaural beats and isochronic tones have been shown to stimulate specific brainwave states (such as theta and delta), which are associated with deep learning, emotional processing, and cellular repair. When paired with hypnosis, these frequencies can open neurological "gateways" for targeted healing.

Unprocessed emotional trauma creates somatic signatures.   Emotional wounds are not "in your head"—they are stored in your body. Studies in trauma neuroscience show that unresolved experiences can dysregulate the hypothalamic-pituitary-adrenal (HPA) axis, increase inflammation, and even alter gene expression. Trauma leaves what we now call somatic imprints, visible through altered neural patterns and chronic symptoms.

Healing as a multidimensional process

We now understand that healing is not just biochemical—it is:

Electrical, driven by neuro-signal patterns and energy fields.

Emotional, shaped by perception, meaning, and memory.

Informational, depending on the quality of instructions received by the brain and body

This insight reframes illness and healing.What was once treated as a breakdown is now understood as a misalignment of information, a loop of outdated signals that hypnosis and neuroplastic interventions can gently interrupt and reprogram.

This scientific awakening is the foundation of the HypnoCell® Method. It is time to move beyond the outdated view of the body as a machine and embrace the reality of the body as an adaptive, intelligent system—one that responds powerfully to directed intention, coherence, and inner alignment.

Introducing Hypnocell®: Healing through neuroplasticity and hypnotic precision

HypnoCell® is a therapeutic methodology born at the intersection of two revolutionary fields: regenerative medicine and clinical hypnosis. It emerged from years of observing what conventional treatments couldn't explain—and what the human body could do when the right mental and biological conditions were created.

At its core, HypnoCell® is built upon a radical but evidence-supported idea: The body is designed to regenerate—but only if the brain believes it is safe to do so.

The foundations of the method

The HypnoCell approach is grounded in three scientific pillars:

Neuroplasticity-   The brain is not hardwired. It constantly reshapes itself through experience, intention, and repetition. Neural pathways—whether they support pain, fear, or healing—are plastic, not permanent. With guided focus, these patterns can be interrupted and rewired.

Hypnosis and the Subconscious Mind-

Clinical hypnosis provides a structured, scientifically validated way to access the subconscious and unconscious levels of the mind—the very domains where automatic behaviors, emotional responses, and internalized beliefs reside. This access allows us to bypass surface-level resistance and work directly with the blueprint that governs biology.

Signal-Based Reframing and Cellular Regeneration-   Every symptom, every emotional or physiological disturbance, carries a message. HypnoCell® is not about "fixing a problem"—it's about decoding that message, identifying the root signal, and creating a new narrative that the nervous system can safely integrate. When the signal changes, so does the biology.

The mechanism: Precision healing through trance

The HypnoCell® process follows a stepwise protocol that leverages the power of the trance state:Induce: A targeted hypnotic induction is used to guide the brain into a reparative state—usually within theta or delta wave frequencies, where deep plasticity and parasympathetic healing occur.

Decode: The subconscious is prompted to surface symbolic or emotional representations of the origin of imbalance—often pre-verbal memories, inherited patterns, or stored trauma responses.

Reframe: Through precision language and imagery, these internal blueprints are gently restructured into patterns of safety, vitality, and coherence.

Embed: The new neural script is installed with multisensory reinforcement, guiding the nervous system to adopt it as a new default response.

Beyond symptoms: The integration of lifestyle and inner alignment

HypnoCell® is not a quick fix—it's a systemic reset. For lasting change, the neural messages must align with the daily signals the body receives. That's why the HypnoCell® method integrates:

Lifestyle modification: Nutrition, rest, movement, and nature are not "wellness extras"—they're biological inputs that influence gene expression and brain chemistry.

Self-hypnosis and meditation: Patients learn to access reparative states on their own, reinforcing the new pathways and becoming active participants in their recovery.

Emotional awareness and narrative repair: Healing isn't only physical—it's also the reclamation of meaning, purpose, and inner safety.

Who this is for?

Whether you are:

A healthcare provider seeking deeper tools to support your patients.

A patient navigating chronic illness, infertility, emotional trauma, or neurological injury.

Or a curious mind looking to understand and harness your brain's innate healing capacity.

...this book will guide you toward a new understanding of healing: one that is grounded in biology, supported by science, and animated by hope and precision.

The body is not broken.

The brain is not static.

Healing is not a mystery—it's a method.

······•··•···

Chapter 1

The brain as an adaptive organ

For much of modern history, the human brain was thought to be a fixed structure—a biological computer with limited capacity, set early in life and destined for decline with age. Brain cells, we were told, don't regenerate. Personality is hardwired. Cognitive functions decline inevitably. Damage is permanent.

We now know these ideas were wrong.

In the last two decades, neuroscience has completely rewritten our understanding of the brain. The brain is not static—it is plastic, meaning it can change its structure and function in response to experience, environment, thought, and intention.

This is not just a poetic metaphor. Neuroplasticity is a measurable biological phenomenon. It is the reason stroke patients can regain function. It is how trauma survivors can rewire fear responses. It is why mindfulness and learning can reshape memory, mood, and even immune function.

To heal, the brain must be flexible. To be flexible, the brain must feel safe.

Understanding how the brain adapts—what conditions enhance or inhibit its regenerative capacity—is the first step toward harnessing its full potential.

From machine to ecosystem

In contrast to the outdated view of the brain as a machine with fixed wiring, modern research reveals it to be more like an ecosystem: constantly shifting, updating, pruning, and reconnecting in response to internal and external signals.

New neurons can be generated (a process known as neurogenesis) in specific areas like the hippocampus.

Synaptic connections can be strengthened or weakened depending on use or disuse.

Emotional, sensory, and cognitive inputs continuously shape network architecture.

This means the brain is not just reactive—it is highly programmable, especially under the right conditions. And when guided intentionally, this adaptability can be used to reverse damage, change behavior, and even support cellular-level repair.

The conditions that shape the brain

The brain's regenerative potential is not evenly distributed or automatic. Neuroplasticity is experience-dependent, and it is influenced by:

Repetition (consistent thought and behavior patterns)

Emotional intensity (strong experiences create deeper imprints)

State of consciousness (trance, meditation, or theta brainwave states enhance rewiring)

Environmental input (nutrition, sleep, stress, sensory stimulation)

Internal belief systems (what the subconscious believes shapes what the body allows)

Hypnosis becomes powerful because it creates an ideal internal environment for plasticity: deep focus, emotional resonance, safety, and suggestibility—all conditions that optimize the brain's receptivity to new patterns.

Your brain is always listening

What you think, say, visualize, and feel—all send signals that your brain translates into chemical and electrical activity. Over time, those patterns become instructions, and those instructions become biology.

This chapter will explore:

How plasticity works at the cellular and network level

The difference between structural and functional changes

How stress and trauma inhibit adaptability

And how you can create the internal environment for your brain to regenerate

Healing begins not when we fight disease, but when we activate the intelligence already built into the nervous system.

Let's begin by understanding the organ that controls it all—not just the brain as we've known it, but the adaptive, intelligent, and rewritable brain we are just beginning to understand.

How the brain changes itself: Neurogenesis, synaptic plasticity, and rewiring

One of the most extraordinary discoveries in modern neuroscience is that the brain is not hardwired—it is dynamic, self-adjusting, and capable of regeneration. Every thought, behavior, experience, and emotional state leaves an imprint on its structure. This ability to change is known as neuroplasticity, and it is the biological foundation for learning, memory, healing, and behavioral transformation.

There are three main mechanisms through which the brain transforms itself:

1. Neurogenesis – Growing new brain cells

For decades, it was believed that we are born with all the brain cells we'll ever have, and that once damaged or lost, neurons could not be replaced. This myth has been firmly debunked.

Research shows that neurogenesis, the birth of new neurons, occurs throughout life—particularly in the hippocampus, a region essential for learning, memory, mood regulation, and stress resilience.

Neurogenesis is influenced by:

Physical exercise (especially aerobic)

Sleep quality

Nutritional factors (omega-3s, polyphenols, curcumin, etc.)

Meditation and mindfulness

Exposure to novelty and learning

States of emotional safety and low chronic stress

What shuts neurogenesis down? Cortisol. Chronic stress, trauma, and unresolved emotional states can inhibit neurogenesis and shrink hippocampal volume over time—often seen in depression, PTSD, and cognitive decline. This is where hypnosis and deep brain relaxation become therapeutic: they lower the stress response and re-open the regenerative window.

2. Synaptic plasticity – Strengthening or weakening neural pathways

Synaptic plasticity refers to the brain's ability to modify the strength and efficiency of communication between neurons. This is the neurobiological basis of learning and habit formation.

There are two key processes:

Long-Term Potentiation (LTP): When a neural pathway is activated repeatedly or emotionally, the connection strengthens—"neurons that fire together wire together."

Long-Term Depression (LTD): When a pathway is unused or inhibited, its strength fades—"neurons that don't fire together, disconnect."

This mechanism explains how we develop automatic patterns, both helpful and harmful:

Chronic fear and worry strengthen anxiety pathways.

Repetitive self-criticism strengthens depressive thinking.

Just as easily, positive visualization, gratitude, and self-compassion can create new, healthier circuits.

Hypnosis works by accessing the subconscious mind where these associations are stored, and reprogramming synaptic pathways with targeted imagery, belief revision, and emotional rewiring.

3. Rewiring – Remapping brain networks

Rewiring refers to large-scale changes in how brain regions coordinate and communicate. This includes:

Functional remapping (e.g., how stroke survivors learn to walk again)

Emotional remapping (changing how memories are processed and stored)

Identity-level shifts (changing the inner narrative that governs self-perception)

Brain networks—like the default mode network (DMN), salience network, and executive control system—are fluid. Their balance determines how we process the world, respond to challenges, and regulate emotions. When trauma, grief, or chronic stress disrupt these networks, we see dysfunction. But when we use tools like hypnosis, meditation, and intentional reframing, these networks can reorganize, creating space for new responses and healing trajectories.

The brain is not a rigid command center—it is a living, learning, and adaptive organ. Through:

Neurogenesis, we grow new capacity.

Synaptic plasticity, we reinforce or release patterns.

Rewiring, we change how the brain operates at scale.

These mechanisms can be consciously activated—especially in the hypnotic state, where the brain becomes most receptive to change.

Understanding these biological truths empowers us to ask a radical question:

What if healing isn't about fighting the body—but about teaching the brain a new way to be?

Brain anatomy 101 for healing

Key regions involved in emotion, trauma, and repair

To understand how hypnosis can influence healing, we must first understand the architecture of the brain—not in exhaustive anatomical detail, but in functional terms: which areas govern our emotions, how trauma is encoded, and where repair processes are regulated.

The human brain is an incredibly complex organ, but when it comes to emotional and physiological healing, a few key structures stand out. These regions form a dynamic network that processes threat, safety, pain, attachment, and ultimately, recovery.

1. The Amygdala – The alarm system

The amygdala is the brain's fear and threat detector. It rapidly processes signals from the senses and decides whether the body should respond with fight, flight, freeze, or fawn. In trauma, the amygdala often becomes hyperactive, interpreting even minor stimuli as threats.

An overactive amygdala leads to:

Chronic stress and anxiety

Hypervigilance

Difficulty relaxing or sleeping

Heightened emotional reactivity

Hypnosis can downregulate amygdala activity, helping shift the nervous system from survival to restoration. This is one of the ways trance states promote safety and neuroregeneration.

2. The Hippocampus – **Memory and context**

Located in the temporal lobe, the hippocampus is responsible for:

Encoding explicit memories

Providing contextual information to emotional experiences

Distinguishing between past and present

Trauma often impairs hippocampal function, which is why past events can feel like they're happening now. In PTSD, for example, the hippocampus fails to "time-stamp" memories, keeping the person in a loop of re-experiencing.

Hypnosis helps by reactivating the hippocampus in a relaxed, plastic state, allowing old experiences to be reprocessed with new meaning and context.

3. The Prefrontal Cortex (PFC) – **Executive control and reappraisal**

The prefrontal cortex is the rational, reflective part of the brain—it evaluates risk, regulates emotions, and suppresses impulses. It also plays a major role in:

Perspective taking

Self-awareness

Goal setting and behavior planning

Chronic stress and trauma can impair PFC function, leading to poor emotional regulation, impulsivity, and difficulty making decisions. In therapeutic hypnosis, PFC activation is modulated, allowing for the integration of new insights and reappraisal of painful events.

4. The Anterior Cingulate Cortex (ACC) – **Emotional regulation and conflict monitoring**

The ACC helps manage emotional pain, self-control, **and** internal conflict. It acts as a bridge between emotion (limbic system) and cognition (PFC), helping the brain resolve "should I vs. want to" dilemmas and recover from emotional distress.

The ACC is also involved in hypnotic suggestibility—research shows greater activity here correlates with responsiveness to hypnosis. When engaged, it helps the brain override habitual responses and adopt new ones.

5. The Insula – **Interoception and mind–body awareness**

The insula processes internal body sensations—heartbeat, breath, pain, temperature, and gut feelings. It's central to interoception, our ability to sense and interpret what's happening inside our bodies.

When trauma disconnects us from bodily awareness, the insula becomes underactive or dysregulated. Hypnosis helps reconnect mind and body, improving sensory integration and somatic awareness, which is essential for restoring homeostasis and self-trust.

6. The Default Mode Network (DMN) – **Inner world and identity**

The DMN is a network of brain regions that activates during rest and self-reflection. It governs:

Internal dialogue

Sense of self and identity

Mental time travel (imagining past/future)

Self-evaluation and meaning-making

In trauma or depression, the DMN can become overactive, creating rumination, self-criticism, and disconnection from the present. In trance states, the DMN's activity often reduces, allowing for a quieting of inner chatter and an opening to deeper, transformative experiences.

Integration: How healing happens across the brain

Healing is not localized to one brain region—it's an orchestrated process involving communication across all these areas. In trauma, these circuits become dysregulated. In hypnosis, we can help restore functional integration—calming overactive circuits and activating underutilized ones.

The HypnoCell® method uses this neuroanatomical understanding to design targeted protocols that speak the brain's language—safety, focus, imagery, rhythm, and suggestion—to create conditions for repair and reprogramming.

When these systems synchronize, the brain no longer sees healing as a risk—it sees it as the natural next step.

What modern neuroscience reveals about self-directed healing

One of the most empowering revelations of modern neuroscience is that healing is not only possible—it can be initiated from within. While external interventions like medications and surgeries have their place, a growing body of evidence now confirms that the mind itself plays a crucial role in determining how the body responds, recovers, and regenerates.

This concept—once dismissed as pseudoscience or "mind over matter" idealism—is now backed by hard data. The brain is not a passive observer in health. It is an active command center capable of influencing every system in the body: the immune response, hormone levels, inflammatory processes, cellular repair, and even gene expression.

The brain's influence on the body

Studies in psychoneuroimmunology, epigenetics, **and** neuroplasticity have shown that:

Thoughts and emotions trigger chemical cascades in the brain that affect everything from heart rate to immune function.

Focused mental states—such as those reached during hypnosis or meditation—alter brainwave activity and shift the nervous system toward healing modes (parasympathetic dominance).

Positive expectations and belief in recovery can increase the effectiveness of treatments (placebo response), reduce pain, and accelerate recovery times.

Mental rehearsal and visualization can activate the same neural pathways as physical action, facilitating motor recovery after injury or stroke.

Subconscious patterns—often formed in childhood or during trauma—can either block or unlock healing, depending on how they are engaged and reprogrammed.

In other words, the brain doesn't just respond to healing—it can initiate it.

Neuroplasticity: The engine of change

At the heart of self-directed healing is neuroplasticity—the brain's ability to change its structure and function in response to experience and intention. This means that with the right internal conditions, the brain can:

Unlearn fear responses and pain associations

Rewire the meaning attached to past events

Downregulate the stress response system (HPA axis)

Reinforce new, health-promoting behaviors and perceptions

Create a fertile internal environment for cellular repair and immune modulation

These are not vague concepts. Brain scans confirm that patients who practice meditation, hypnosis, or mental visualization show measurable changes in gray matter density, neural connectivity, and emotional regulation networks.

Healing is an information-based process

Modern neuroscience is also reframing our understanding of healing as an informational process—not just a mechanical or biochemical one.

Every organ, tissue, and cell in the body operates through communication: electrical impulses, chemical messengers, and signaling proteins. These systems are influenced not only by external factors (like medication), but by internal perception and meaning.

When you shift what you believe about your illness—when you feel safe, empowered, supported—your nervous system sends a different signal to your cells. Stress chemicals like cortisol decrease. Inflammatory markers drop. Growth factors increase. The immune system recalibrates. Tissue repair begins.

This is why chronic stress, unprocessed trauma, or a belief that "I will never heal" can become biological barriers to recovery.

Conversely, when the brain receives new instructions—through hypnosis, imagery, or belief revision—it updates the body accordingly. This is self-directed healing in action.

A therapeutic revolution

We are now in the midst of a quiet revolution in medicine—one where healing is not seen as something done to the body, but as something co-created with the mind. Hypnosis is not a trick; it is a tool. And neuroplasticity is not a miracle; it is a mechanism.

The implications are vast:

Patients can learn to regulate their own physiology.

Chronic pain can be reduced without drugs.

Emotional trauma can be reframed at the neural level.

Recovery can be accelerated by changing internal narratives and perceptions.

The HypnoCell® Method is built on this understanding. It offers structured, scientific pathways to access the brain's healing systems through precision hypnosis, subconscious rewiring, and neuro-regenerative guidance.

Healing is not something we wait for.It's something we can help the brain choose.

· · · · ● · ● · · · ·

Chapter 2
Mapping the mind

Concious, subconcious and unconcious layers

To understand how hypnosis can lead to healing and reprogramming, we must first understand how the human mind is organized. Much like the layers of an operating system, the mind is composed of distinct levels, each with unique functions, access points, and influence over health and behavior.

Modern psychology, neuroscience, and hypnosis research have helped us refine what early thinkers like Freud, Jung, and Janet theorized: that the mind is not a single entity, but a layered system, where the majority of our biological and behavioral programming occurs beneath the surface of conscious awareness.

Let's explore these layers:

1. The Conscious Mind – **The tip of the iceberg**

The conscious mind is the smallest, but most visible part of our mental activity. It represents what we are aware of in the present moment—logical thought, rational decision-making, focus, and voluntary actions.

Functions include:

Analytical thinking

Goal setting

Temporary memory

Judgments and reasoning

Awareness of the current environment

Despite its importance, the conscious mind processes only about 40–50 bits of information per second, while the subconscious handles millions. This is why attempts to "will" ourselves into health, change, or calmness often fail. The conscious mind may want healing—but the deeper systems must believe it is safe.

2. The Subconscious Mind – **The control center**

Beneath conscious awareness lies the subconscious mind, a vast system responsible for:

Emotional responses

Learned behaviors and habits

Memory storage

Language associations

Bodily functions (breathing, digestion, hormone regulation)

It acts like an autopilot system, driving over 90% of our daily behaviors, choices, and biological processes. It is non-linear, emotional, and symbolic—responding best to imagery, repetition, suggestion, and emotional resonance.

Importantly, the subconscious does not distinguish between real and imagined experience. That's why hypnosis, visualization, and guided imagery can have measurable physiological effects: when done correctly, the subconscious accepts these inputs as "real" and adjusts bodily systems accordingly.

When trauma, chronic stress, or negative beliefs get encoded here, they shape the body's response: immune suppression, muscle tension, inflammation, hormonal imbalances, even infertility. But when new instructions are delivered in a receptive state—such as hypnosis—the subconscious can accept, reframe, and reprogram.

3. The Unconscious Mind – The deep archive

The unconscious is the deepest and most inaccessible part of the mind. It stores:

Pre-verbal experiences

Suppressed memories

Instincts and survival patterns

Ancestral and inherited imprints (epigenetic influence)

Collective symbols and archetypes (Jungian theory)

Though not directly accessible through ordinary awareness, the unconscious shapes the foundation of identity, drives compulsions, and influences cellular memory. It's also where trauma that bypassed verbal processing often resides.

Hypnosis is one of the few tools that can bridge into the unconscious, using metaphor, archetype, and deep-trance techniques to retrieve, recontextualize, and transform these latent patterns.

Interaction between layers

These three layers do not operate independently—they interact continuously, forming what we call the "mind-body loop":

A thought in the conscious mind triggers an emotion in the subconscious, which can activate an autonomic response rooted in the unconscious.

Conversely, a body sensation or emotional flashback can surface from the unconscious through the subconscious, eventually reaching the conscious mind as anxiety, a limiting belief, or unexplained pain.

Healing becomes sustainable only when all three layers are aligned. That means:

The conscious mind understands the issue.

The subconscious mind feels safe to change.

The unconscious mind is heard, seen, and updated with new information.

HypnoCell® and the mind map

The HypnoCell® method uses this layered model to:

Induce access to subconscious and unconscious material.

Decode symbolic language used by the deeper mind.

Deliver new instructions through imagery, suggestion, and emotional repair.

Synchronize the layers, so biology follows updated beliefs and inner safety.

When these systems communicate harmoniously, the nervous system can release survival mode, inflammation can calm, and regenerative processes can begin.

Healing happens at the speed of alignment—not force.

Functional roles of each level of awareness

To create lasting healing, transformation must occur across all levels of the mind—not just intellectually, but emotionally, biologically, and symbolically. Each level of awareness—the conscious, subconscious, and unconscious—has a distinct functional role in shaping perception, behavior, emotion, and physiology.

Understanding how these layers work individually—and in collaboration—is central to applying the HypnoCell® method for neuroplastic healing.

1. The Conscious Mind

Role: Awareness, Evaluation, and Short-Term Decision Making.

The conscious mind is the part we use to observe, plan, analyze, and respond in real time. It is:

Rational and analytical

Goal-directed

Responsible for immediate attention and thought

Closely linked to our sense of identity and agency

Strengths:

Can override automatic reactions (with effort)

Helps us make sense of past and future

Drives intentional change and behavior modification (temporarily)

Limitations:

Processes a limited amount of data per second (~40–50 bits)

Easily overwhelmed by emotional overload

Has little direct influence over autonomic functions (e.g., heart rate, hormone output)

In healing: The conscious mind is useful for setting intentions, understanding patterns, and initiating change—but it cannot do the heavy lifting alone.

2. The Subconscious Mind

Role: Emotion, Habit, Memory, and Biological Regulation

The subconscious is the emotional and sensory warehouse of your mind. It governs:

Stored memories and past experiences

Emotional responses (especially conditioned ones)

Beliefs, habits, and learned behaviors

Physical processes like digestion, immune function, hormone secretion

Strengths:

Can process millions of bits of information per second

Functions autonomously—keeps us alive and functioning

Responds deeply to repetition, imagery, emotion, and suggestion

Limitations:

Is non-logical and cannot reason like the conscious mind

Accepts experiences and messages as "truth," especially if emotional

Cannot distinguish between real and imagined inputs

In healing: The subconscious is the target of hypnosis—it holds the patterns that drive biological responses. By communicating directly with it, we can reshape how the body responds to stress, pain, inflammation, and cellular repair.

3. The Unconscious Mind

Role: Instinct, Identity Imprints, and Deep Survival Programming

The unconscious mind is the deepest layer, often inaccessible through logic or language. It stores:

Pre-verbal, developmental, or even ancestral material

Core identity patterns

Somatic memories and trauma

Survival strategies and primal instincts

Strengths:

Protects the organism at all costs

Governs fight-flight-freeze responses

Holds symbolic content and powerful archetypes

Often the true source of "mystery illnesses" or stuck emotional patterns

Limitations:

Cannot be accessed directly through conscious effort

Speaks in symbols, metaphors, and dreams—not words

Operates reactively unless updated

In healing: When trauma, emotional shock, or chronic fear is stored here, it drives unconscious resistance to healing. HypnoCell® uses trance states and symbolic language to gently surface and integrate these imprints, allowing for reorganization of deeply embedded responses.

Why integration matters

These levels of awareness work best when they are aligned. Healing becomes difficult when:

The conscious mind wants change,

But the subconscious still fears it,

And the unconscious has encoded it as dangerous.

In this mismatch, the nervous system prioritizes survival over repair—even if the threat is no longer real.

HypnoCell® works by:

Helping the conscious mind gain insight and clarity

Guiding the subconscious mind into plastic, receptive states

Gently decoding and updating unconscious material through suggestion, metaphor, and symbolic processing.

When awareness is layered, healing is partial. When awareness is integrated, healing is exponential.

How healing must involve the subconscious and unconscious to be lasting

In clinical medicine, we often define healing as the resolution of symptoms. Pain is gone. Inflammation is reduced. Fertility returns. A scan is clear.

But from a neurobiological and mind–body perspective, true healing is not just the removal of symptoms—it is the restoration of internal safety, coherence, and adaptability. And that kind of transformation cannot happen solely through conscious effort. It must involve the subconscious and unconscious layers of the mind, where the patterns that drive biology are stored.

Why surface-level healing often fails

Many patients seek help for symptoms that seem to resolve temporarily—only to return weeks, months, or years later. This is especially common in chronic fatigue, anxiety, trauma responses, hormonal dysfunction, autoimmune flares, or infertility. They may have tried diet changes, medications, supplements, talk therapy, and mindset work, yet the shifts don't stick.

Why?

Because while the conscious mind may want change, the deeper layers of the mind—the subconscious and unconscious—still perceive the change as unsafe.

When unresolved experiences, survival responses, or limiting beliefs are held beneath awareness, they act as a biological override, continually signaling the nervous system to:

Stay in fight or flight

Suppress immune and reproductive functions

Remain hypervigilant or emotionally frozen

Block receptivity to repair, intimacy, or expansion

Until these signals are decoded and updated, the body resists full recovery. The deeper mind always wins.

The Subconscious: Where Patterns Live

The subconscious mind governs:

Conditioned emotional responses

Habits and identity beliefs

Autonomic functions (heartbeat, hormones, immunity)

Stored memory associations (often linked to trauma or shame)

This level operates like a software program—it runs silently in the background, directing behavior and physiology based on what it believes is true.

In cases of chronic illness or emotional blocks, the subconscious may have encoded messages like:

"It's not safe to let go."

"Healing means vulnerability."

"I don't deserve to be well."

"If I'm healthy, I'll be abandoned."

No supplement or conscious mantra can override these deeply embedded patterns. But hypnosis can access and reprogram them, often quickly and with long-term impact—because it speaks the language of the subconscious: imagery, feeling, repetition, and suggestion.

The Unconscious: Where Survival Lives

The unconscious mind holds:

Preverbal trauma

Somatic memory (the body's memory)

Instinctual responses and primal fears

Inherited emotional coding (epigenetics, family systems)

This level is responsible for the deepest survival patterns, and it is highly symbolic. A person may not consciously remember what shaped their illness or block, but the unconscious holds the imprint—in a sensation, image, or archetype.

Through deep-trance work and metaphor, HypnoCell® reaches into these buried layers, allowing the unconscious to safely:

Surface what was once too overwhelming to process

Re-interpret it with new meaning

Release the survival pattern that no longer serves

Restore nervous system equilibrium

The missing link in most treatments

This is why treatments that focus only on symptoms or conscious behavior change often fail to deliver permanent results. They don't reach the inner programs that drive biology and behavior.

When healing is only conscious, the nervous system may remain dysregulated.

When healing is subconscious and unconscious, the nervous system can finally relax.

In that state of deep safety, plasticity is activated, immune function improves, hormones recalibrate, and tissue can regenerate.

This is where HypnoCell® offers its most powerful impact: not through suggestion alone, but by restoring communication between mind, body, and biology at every level of awareness.

You cannot heal the body while the subconscious mind still believes you're in danger.

And you cannot override unconscious imprints without accessing their language.

True healing requires full-system alignment.

Why conscious willpower is not enough

"Just think positive."

"Try harder."

"Be more disciplined."

"Mind over matter."

These are common refrains in the self-help world and even in some therapeutic settings. While well-intentioned, these statements reflect a fundamental misunderstanding of how the human mind and body operate. They assume that the conscious mind is in control—that if we simply decide to change, our thoughts and behaviors will follow.

But neuroscience tells a different story.

The conscious mind, responsible for logic, analysis, and decision-making, governs only about 5–10% of our cognitive activity. The remaining 90–95% is subconscious or unconscious, driven by deeply ingrained emotional patterns, beliefs, memories, and physiological states that operate beneath awareness.

This is why willpower alone often fails—especially in the face of:

Chronic illness

Emotional trauma

Addictions and compulsions

Infertility or hormonal imbalances

Anxiety, depression, or self-sabotage

These challenges are not rooted in laziness, weakness, or lack of motivation. They are embedded in automatic programs running beneath the surface.

The limits of the "Thinking Brain"

The prefrontal cortex, the seat of willpower, is easily overpowered when:

Stress levels are high

Emotions are intense

Old trauma is triggered

The body is in survival mode (fight, flight, freeze, or fawn)

In these states, the brain defaults to older, faster systems—the limbic system and brainstem—which are not rational but reactive. These areas prioritize protection, not progress.

So even when a person consciously wants to change, heal, or move forward, their deeper mind may be running protective scripts such as:

"It's safer to stay where I am."

"If I change, I might get hurt again."

"Being ill gives me identity, connection, or control."

"Healing would force me to face a truth I'm not ready for."

These scripts are not accessible through conscious logic—but they can be accessed and reprogrammed through hypnosis and subconscious work.

Willpower vs. subconscious conditioning

Here's a metaphor to illustrate the imbalance:

Imagine trying to steer a boat with a tiny rudder (your conscious mind) while the engine (your subconscious) is set on full speed in the opposite direction. You may hold the rudder tightly and exert effort, but unless the engine's course is changed, you will constantly struggle, drift, or burn out.

Lasting healing requires changing the direction of the engine—not just gripping the rudder harder.

That's why:

Telling someone with trauma to "just move on" doesn't work.

Repeating affirmations without emotional integration feels hollow.

Trying to control symptoms without addressing the emotional imprint leads to relapse.

The solution: Access and align the deeper mind

To create lasting change, we must:

Access the subconscious patterns driving the body's responses.

Identify and update the emotional associations and beliefs encoded in the nervous system.

Align the conscious intention with subconscious safety and unconscious permission.

This is what the HypnoCell® Method is designed to do:It bypasses the critical, surface-level mind and goes straight to the source—the patterns that govern biology, emotion, and behavior.

By using clinical hypnosis and guided neuroplastic techniques, we don't force change through effort—we invite transformation through internal realignment.

Willpower may initiate change.

But only subconscious integration can sustain it.

When the deeper mind agrees, change becomes effortless—and healing becomes inevitable.

·· · ●·●·● ·· ·

Chapter 3

From root signals to regeneration

Healing does not begin with suppressing symptoms—it begins with understanding them. In the HypnoCell® model, what we traditionally call a "problem" is reframed as a root signal: a meaningful message from the body's inner intelligence, expressing itself through discomfort, dysfunction, or dis-ease. These signals often originate from subconscious emotional imprints, unresolved stress, or outdated neural programs—none of which are accessible through logic or willpower alone.

Rather than viewing the body as broken, we approach it as misinformed—caught in a loop of protective patterns that were once useful, but are now limiting regeneration.

This chapter explores how these signals form, how they affect the brain-body system, and how they can be decoded and transformed into pathways for true healing.

Through precision hypnosis, subconscious reprogramming, and emotional resolution, we shift the body's internal language from survival to restoration.

Decoding biological messages for lasting healing

In conventional medicine, symptoms are often treated as errors to be suppressed. Pain is dulled. Hormones are replaced. Inflammation is reduced. While these interventions can provide temporary relief, they frequently fail to address the underlying cause—the signal that gave rise to the symptom in the first place.

In the HypnoCell® method, we view the body not as malfunctioning, but as communicating. Every symptom is seen as a root signal—a bio-intelligent message from the subconscious or unconscious mind, expressed through the nervous system and physiology.

What we call a "problem" may actually be a pattern asking to be heard.

By decoding these signals and guiding the mind into reparative states, we can begin the process of regeneration—not just suppression.

What are root signals?

A root signal is a persistent message encoded in the mind-body system. It may arise from:

Unresolved emotional trauma

Chronic stress patterns

Suppressed memories

Misaligned beliefs about the body, identity, or safety

Pre-verbal or inherited imprints (epigenetic stress memory)

Repetitive negative self-talk or internal conflict

These signals don't only live in the brain—they become embodied, influencing heart rate, hormone levels, digestion, immune response, and more. Over time, they may manifest as chronic symptoms, infertility, autoimmune disease, or fatigue—not because the body is failing, but because it is trying to maintain survival under outdated conditions.

The brain—body loop

When the subconscious perceives an unresolved threat (emotional, relational, existential), it sends ongoing messages to the autonomic nervous system and tissues:

"Hold tension here."

"Suppress reproductive function until it's safe."

"Store energy; don't repair."

"Stay on alert. Don't rest."

Even when the external threat is long gone, the internal program persists, keeping the body in a state of vigilance, inflammation, or shutdown.

This is where HypnoCell® becomes vital: it interrupts the loop, identifies the original signal, and provides the brain with updated instructions aligned with safety, vitality, and restoration.

Reframing the "problem" as information

In HypnoCell, we no longer ask:

"How do we get rid of this pain?"

"How do we silence this symptom?"

We ask:

"What is this signal trying to tell us?"

"What conditions are required for this pattern to resolve itself?"

"What was never processed—and how can we complete it safely now?"

This shift reframes disease as a miscommunication, not a malfunction.

Instead of fighting the body, we listen, decode, and collaborate with its intelligence.

Regeneration begins with resolution

Once the signal is acknowledged, understood, and resolved at the subconscious or unconscious level, the body naturally shifts toward:

Parasympathetic dominance (rest, digest, repair)

Improved neurochemical balance (serotonin, dopamine, oxytocin)

Cellular repair and regeneration (via immune and hormonal recalibration)

Rewiring of stress patterns in the brain and nervous system

This is not forced healing. It is reinstated healing—a return to what the body was designed to do, once the interference is removed.

The HypnoCell® protocol: From signal to safety

In practice, the HypnoCell® process follows four phases:

Access the altered state through trance and relaxation

Identify the root signal: memory, emotion, belief, or sensation

Reframe the pattern through subconscious suggestion, imagery, and integration

Reinforce the new state using repetition, self-hypnosis, and aligned lifestyle signals

This allows the nervous system to stop reacting to the past—and start rebuilding for the present.

Regeneration is not something we force into the body.

It is something we invite, once the signals of threat have been replaced with signals of safety, permission, and repair.

Understanding dysfunction as an informational mismatch, not a "problem"

In traditional medicine, dysfunction is often treated as a problem to be solved, a biological error to be corrected. A symptom is something to suppress. An illness is something to fight. But this framework, while useful in acute care, is fundamentally limiting when applied to chronic, emotional, or stress-related conditions.

In the HypnoCell® model, we replace the concept of "problem" with a more accurate, compassionate, and functional view: dysfunction is an informational mismatch.

The body isn't failing—it's responding to the wrong data.

What is an informational mismatch?

Every cell in the body is influenced by signals it receives from the brain and nervous system. These signals are shaped by:

Emotion

Memory

Perception

Beliefs

Environmental cues

Unconscious safety assessments

When these signals are accurate, the body functions efficiently—adapting, healing, repairing, and regulating itself as needed.

But when the brain is operating on outdated or distorted information, such as:

"I'm still in danger" (from past trauma)

"I'm not safe to rest"

"I must stay alert to survive"

"Healing is unsafe, unfamiliar, or undeserved"

...the result is a physiological response mismatched to the current reality.

This mismatch may present as:

Chronic pain in the absence of tissue damage

Hormonal suppression in the absence of threat

Infertility despite normal reproductive anatomy

Anxiety, fatigue, insomnia, or autoimmunity without a clear cause

These are not errors. They are adaptive responses to perceived input—often originating at the subconscious or unconscious level.

The body responds to perception, not just reality

The nervous system does not wait for conscious thought to decide how to respond. It reacts to subconscious and unconscious cues, many of which were formed early in life, inherited epigenetically, or shaped by emotionally charged experiences.

For example:

A person who grew up in chaos may subconsciously associate peace with danger.

A patient who had a traumatic medical experience may associate healing with threat.

A body conditioned to "perform to be loved" may resist rest or softness, even when it's needed.

These belief-perception loops drive behavior, hormone output, immune modulation, and nervous system tone. The body acts accordingly—not based on logic, but based on what the deeper mind believes to be true.

Reframing dysfunction as feedback

When we stop calling symptoms "problems" and begin to view them as intelligent feedback, everything changes:

We stop fighting our bodies.

We stop fearing our patterns.

We start listening—with precision and compassion.

Symptoms become invitations to decode, reframe, and respond with new information. And this is where HypnoCell® becomes a powerful intervention: it helps identify the mismatch, deliver updated instructions, and re-establish alignment between perception and physiology.

Dysfunction is not failure.

It is feedback.

The body is not broken—it's confused.

Healing begins with clarity.

The body as a messenger: How symptoms reflect unresolved neural patterns

What if symptoms were not malfunctions—but messages?

This simple but powerful question is at the core of the HypnoCell® approach. In conventional medicine, symptoms are often viewed as problems to eliminate. But in reality, they are the body's language—its way of communicating that something in the system is misaligned, incomplete, or unresolved.

In the context of neuroscience and psychobiology, symptoms are not random. They are expressions of unresolved neural patterns—recurring loops within the brain and nervous system that haven't yet been completed, processed, or reframed.

The body doesn't forget—it repeats

The human nervous system is designed for efficiency. Once it learns how to respond to a stimulus—whether physical, emotional, or environmental—it stores that pattern for future use. This is how habits, reflexes, and emotional reactions form.

But what happens when the stored pattern was formed during trauma, prolonged stress, or a misinterpreted threat?

It gets memorized and reinforced, even if the original danger has long passed. The nervous system, in an effort to protect, keeps replaying the same loop:

The heart races in a calm room.

The gut flares in the absence of actual food sensitivity.

Hormones shut down in the presence of unresolved grief.

A fertile body won't conceive while carrying a subconscious imprint of unsafety.

These responses are not irrational—they are misdirected protective strategies, encoded into neural circuits that fire automatically, without conscious awareness.

From signal to symptom: How neural patterns become physical

When a neural loop is repeatedly activated, it begins to shape the entire neurophysiological system:

Emotional Pattern → Fear, guilt, sadness, hypervigilance

Neurological Response → Increased limbic activation (e.g., amygdala), reduced prefrontal regulation

Hormonal and Autonomic Shift → Dysregulation of cortisol, adrenaline, or reproductive hormones

Immune and Inflammatory Output → Chronic low-grade inflammation, pain, autoimmune markers

Tissue-Level Expression → Fatigue, migraines, infertility, digestive issues, chronic tension, etc.

This is not speculation. It is documented in the fields of psychoneuroimmunology and trauma neuroscience. The body holds what the brain doesn't resolve—and it speaks through symptoms.

Common examples of the body as a messenger

Chronic Pain may reflect unresolved grief or suppressed anger held in the muscles and fascia.

Digestive Issues (IBS, nausea, bloating) often reflect subconscious issues with control, shame, or boundary violations.

Infertility can stem from subconscious beliefs of unworthiness, inherited trauma, or fear of motherhood.

Autoimmune Flare-ups frequently follow periods of emotional suppression or identity crisis.

Fatigue or Brain Fog may emerge from years of hyperarousal and adrenal overcompensation.

In each case, the body is not failing—it is communicating. When conventional approaches silence these signals without understanding them, they may reappear elsewhere—or intensify.

HypnoCell®: Listening and rewriting the loop

The HypnoCell® method doesn't ask, "How do we fix the body?"

It asks, "What is the body trying to tell us—and what pattern is it asking us to resolve?"

Through hypnosis and guided neural rewiring, we can:

Access the subconscious loop behind the symptom.

Identify the emotional or perceptual distortion that created the signal.

Reframe the memory, belief, or image at the root.

Install new instructions that align the nervous system with safety and regeneration.

When the loop is completed—when the message is heard and integrated—the symptom often diminishes or disappears, not because it was suppressed, but because its purpose was fulfilled.

The body is not the enemy.

The symptom is not the threat.

Both are guides, pointing us back to what needs resolution.

The HypnoCell® process of tracing back to the originating imprint

Accessing the core signal beneath the symptom:

One of the defining principles of the HypnoCell® method is that symptoms are not random—they are the surface expressions of an underlying imprint.

This imprint is not simply a memory or a belief. It is a neurological and emotional encoding formed at a specific point in time—often during a moment of emotional intensity, trauma, relational rupture, or perceived danger. When that moment goes unresolved, its energetic and neurological signature gets stored in the subconscious or unconscious mind and begins shaping the body's responses.

The body remembers.

The nervous system adapts.

The imprint persists—until it is seen, reframed, and updated.

What is an "Originating Imprint"?

An originating imprint is a core emotional-neural pattern that created a loop in the brain–body system. It typically forms:

During early childhood, when the brain is highly plastic and dependent on safety cues from caregivers.

In moments of intense emotion, when the subconscious is most impressionable.

When the system cannot process or integrate an experience, leading to stored, frozen responses.

Through repetition of stressful experiences, reinforcing maladaptive wiring.

Examples of originating imprints include:

"If I rest, I'll be punished."

"It's dangerous to be seen."

"I must protect others to be loved."

"Healing would make me vulnerable again."

"Being sick keeps me safe, connected, or worthy."

These are not logical beliefs—they are embodied truths for the nervous system, often encoded without words, but stored in sensations, images, and affective tone.

How HypnoCell® locates the imprint

The HypnoCell® method uses hypnosis to bypass the critical conscious mind and gain direct access to the subconscious and unconscious archives. Through a structured process of deep focus, relaxation, and symbolic inquiry, the practitioner or individual can:

Induce a trance state conducive to theta and delta brainwave activity—where the mind becomes open, suggestible, and internally focused.

Invite the symptom to speak through metaphor, sensation, or imagery.

Trace emotional associations back to their earliest, clearest origin—often via regression, body memory, or spontaneous symbolic recall.

Identify the moment of imprint—not to re-traumatize, but to observe it with new understanding, emotional neutrality, and perspective.

This process is trauma-informed and gentle. The goal is not catharsis or emotional overwhelm, but integration—bringing coherence and updated information to a frozen circuit in the system.

Completing the loop to enable regeneration

Once the imprint is located, HypnoCell® guides the mind to:

Reframe the meaning of the event or belief.

Install a new emotional response using visualization, somatic cues, and positive suggestion.

Signal safety to the nervous system through rhythmic breathing, neuro-associative anchoring, and guided sensory imagery.

Encode the new pattern through repetition and post-session reinforcement (e.g., self-hypnosis, meditation, lifestyle alignment).

The shift may not always be dramatic—but it is foundational. With the original imprint transformed, the nervous system no longer needs to generate the symptom as a form of protection, communication, or control. This is when regeneration begins—naturally, biologically, and sustainably.

Why the origin matters

Many therapies focus on symptom management or surface-level mindset work. While helpful, these approaches often miss the root. Unless the originating imprint is located and resolved, the body continues to respond as if the past is still present.

The HypnoCell® process does not aim to fix the body. It creates the conditions for the brain and body to:

Feel safe

Update internal narratives

Restore balance

And return to their innate regenerative intelligence

When we trace the symptom to its source,We don't just relieve suffering—We free the system to evolve.

Emotional resonance, trauma loops, and cellular memory

How unresolved experience echoes through the brain and body.

The human body is not just a biological machine—it's also an emotional archive. Every emotionally charged experience, especially those involving fear, loss, shame, or helplessness, leaves an imprint not only on the mind but also on the nervous system, hormones, muscles, and even gene expression.

Modern neuroscience and trauma research confirm what many healing traditions have long known: when emotional experiences are left unresolved, they do not simply vanish—they become embedded in neural circuits, body systems, and behavior patterns. Over time, this unresolved content contributes to chronic symptoms, stress-related conditions, and emotional dysregulation.

Emotional resonance: When experience gets "stamped" into the system

Emotions are not abstract—they're chemical, electrical, and deeply physical. When an event is emotionally significant, the brain responds by:

Releasing neurochemicals (e.g., cortisol, adrenaline, oxytocin).

Activating specific neural networks (e.g., the amygdala, hippocampus, and insula).

Imprinting the experience through vivid memory, bodily sensations, or behavioral conditioning.

This process is known as emotional encoding or resonance. It helps us learn from experience. But if the emotion is intense and the experience remains unprocessed, the resonance becomes a persistent filter—shaping how we interpret the world, respond to triggers, and regulate our health.

For example:

A person with unresolved betrayal may overreact to harmless interpersonal cues.

A history of powerlessness may show up as chronic tension or pain.

Shame may become embedded in posture, breathing, or digestive function.

These emotional residues linger and shape physiology, even when the conscious mind has moved on.

Trauma loops: Repetition of the unfinished response

When the nervous system encounters overwhelming stress and cannot fully process it—either because the event was too intense, too prolonged, or occurred in a state of powerlessness—it stores the experience as an open loop.

That loop can manifest as:

Persistent emotional reactivity

Anxiety or hypervigilance

Avoidance or emotional shutdown

Patterns of self-sabotage or isolation

Physical symptoms with no clear medical cause

In neuroscience, this is described as abnormal persistence of a survival response—the brain is caught in the past, responding to the present as if it were dangerous.

Trauma loops are not limited to extreme events; they can be formed by:

Repeated emotional invalidation

Chronic stress during early development

Emotional neglect

Cultural or inherited patterns of suppression

To complete the loop, the nervous system must be guided back into a state where it can safely process what was previously overwhelming, often through relaxation, embodiment, and emotional reintegration.

Cellular memory: The body's silent archive

The body stores memory in more than the brain. Research in fields like psychoneuroimmunology and epigenetics shows that chronic stress and unprocessed emotion can alter:

Immune function

Gene expression

Hormone sensitivity

Tissue inflammation

Muscle tone and posture

This is known as cellular memory—the idea that the body "remembers" through its cells, tissues, and regulatory systems. It explains why someone may feel unexplained fear or pain in the absence of external threat: their internal landscape is still carrying the imprint of the past.

Cellular memory is not mystical—it is measurable. For instance:

People with PTSD often show changes in immune markers and cortisol rhythms.

Early life adversity correlates with chronic disease risk decades later.

Emotions like grief or resentment, when unexpressed, are associated with specific organ system patterns (e.g., tension in the chest, gut, or pelvis).

Releasing the past to reset the system

For healing to be complete—not just symptom-based—it must include the release or resolution of these unresolved emotional imprints.

This often involves:

Accessing deep states of calm and introspection (e.g., meditation, trance, deep relaxation).

Allowing emotional content to emerge safely and without judgment.

Completing old survival responses (e.g., shaking, crying, breathwork).

Updating the nervous system with new signals of safety and self-agency.

When this happens, emotional resonance fades, trauma loops dissolve, and the body stops reacting to an outdated narrative. The shift may be subtle or profound—but it always begins with recognizing that symptoms are not failures. They are echoes. Messages. Opportunities for resolution.

The mind may forget.

But the body remembers—until it's given permission to release.

Healing begins when the past no longer shapes the present.

Chapter 4

The frequency code - healing through vibrations

How sound, rhythm, and brainwaves can rewire the mind and body.

We Are Frequency.

We often think of the body in biochemical terms—hormones, enzymes, neurotransmitters. But beneath that chemistry lies an even more fundamental layer: electrical signaling and vibrational frequency. Every cell in your body communicates not only through molecules, but through energy—oscillations, impulses, rhythms.

The heart emits electromagnetic fields measurable several feet from the body. The brain pulses with waves of electrical activity that shift according to state of consciousness. Bones, organs, and even DNA resonate at specific frequencies. In fact, all living tissues vibrate, and this vibration plays a role in health, communication, and even repair.

Healing, then, is not only a chemical event.It is also an energetic correction, a tuning of a system that has fallen out of coherence.

In this chapter, we'll explore how vibration and frequency—through sound, rhythm, and brainwave entrainment—can support healing, enhance neuroplasticity, and open access to subconscious and unconscious layers of the mind. This is what we call the frequency code: a set of biological and energetic principles through which the body re-learns how to regulate, restore, and regenerate.

Brainwave states: The gateways of consciousness

The brain operates at different frequencies depending on your mental and emotional state. These frequencies are known as brainwaves, and they correspond to how alert, focused, creative, or relaxed you are:

Beta (13–30 Hz) – Waking consciousness, focused thinking, stress response

Alpha (8–12 Hz) – Relaxed focus, calm alertness, flow states

Theta (4–7 Hz) – Dreamlike states, deep meditation, subconscious access

Delta (0.5–4 Hz) – Deep sleep, regeneration, unconscious processing

Gamma (30+ Hz) – High-level problem solving, insight, and integrative thinking

Theta and delta waves, in particular, are highly regenerative. These are the frequencies where:

Memory reconsolidation occurs

Emotional integration is possible

Healing hormones are released

The immune system reboots

These states are naturally reached in deep meditation, sleep, and hypnosis. But they can also be intentionally induced—a process known as entrainment.

Brainwave entrainment: Tuning the mind for change

Brainwave entrainment is the use of external rhythmic stimuli—typically sound—to synchronize brainwave activity to a desired frequency. This can be achieved through:

Binaural beats – Different tones played in each ear, producing a perceived third frequency.

Isochronic tones – Single tones turned on and off at precise intervals.

Rhythmic drumming or sound therapy – Ancient methods shown to shift consciousness.

When the brain receives repeated, rhythmic input, it naturally begins to match the frequency—a phenomenon called the frequency following response. This allows us to shift into states that support healing, learning, and integration.

Clinical studies show that entrainment can:

Reduce anxiety and cortisol levels

Improve focus and sleep quality

Facilitate trauma resolution

Enhance responsiveness to therapeutic suggestions

The body as a resonant system

Every organ, tissue, and cell resonates at its own natural frequency. When exposed to frequencies that are harmonious or restorative, the body can:

Relax into parasympathetic dominance

Decrease inflammation

Improve cellular coherence (measured through heart rate variability and EEG)

Reconnect disrupted energy patterns (as measured in functional MRI and biofield studies)

Some researchers and practitioners refer to this as vibrational medicine. While still controversial in conventional circles, the growing body of research suggests that frequency-based interventions—including sound baths, voice toning, pulsed electromagnetic fields, and light therapies—can promote measurable biological shifts.

Why frequency matters in healing

The nervous system is especially sensitive to rhythmic input. This is why certain sounds can make us feel safe, soothed, or deeply introspective, while others can agitate or overwhelm. In healing contexts, frequency becomes a carrier of safety, meaning, and neuroplastic opportunity.

When the right frequency is combined with intention and emotional resonance, the body becomes:

More receptive to change

Less guarded against past patterns

Better able to access deeper levels of consciousness where true rewiring occurs

This is why frequency work is often paired with hypnosis, breathwork, meditation, or trauma therapy—because it opens the door for the nervous system to receive and integrate new information without resistance.

Integration: Applying the frequency code

To integrate frequency into healing, consider:

Using theta and delta soundscapes before or during self-hypnosis or inner work.

Practicing rhythmic breathing (coherent breathing at ~5–6 breaths per minute) to entrain heart and brain rhythms.

Exploring guided audio programs designed to regulate vagal tone and brainwave balance.

Reducing exposure to chaotic sensory inputs (noise pollution, digital overstimulation) that disrupt internal rhythm.

When used skillfully, frequency is not just calming—it is transformative. It creates the conditions in which the mind relaxes, the body recalibrates, and healing becomes possible from the inside out.

We are not just flesh and bone.

We are rhythm and resonance.

To heal the body, sometimes we must first tune the frequency.

Brainwaves and their healing potential

Tapping into the natural frequencies of the mind

The human brain is a dynamic electrical organ. Every second, billions of neurons are firing, communicating through tiny bursts of electricity. This electrical activity produces brainwaves, which can be measured in Hertz (cycles per second) using an EEG (electroencephalogram).

Different brainwave frequencies correspond to different states of consciousness, awareness, and physiological function. Importantly, each of these states plays a unique role in the brain's ability to regulate the body, process emotions, store memories, and promote healing.

Understanding how these frequencies work—and how to access them—provides one of the most powerful tools for self-directed healing, mental reprogramming, and nervous system regulation.

Delta Waves (0.5–4 Hz)

The deep healing state

Delta is the slowest brainwave frequency and is dominant during deep, dreamless sleep. It is also present during the most profound states of trance, unconsciousness, and physical repair.

Associated with:

Deep physical regeneration and cellular repair

Release of growth hormone and immune regulation

Restorative sleep and detoxification

Access to the unconscious mind and primal memories

Delta waves are crucial for body repair, especially during non-REM sleep stages. Disrupted delta activity has been linked to chronic fatigue, fibromyalgia, immune dysfunction, and poor stress resilience.

Some advanced meditative states and deep hypnosis sessions can access delta, allowing the nervous system to shift into a profound parasympathetic state, where true regeneration can occur.

Theta Waves (4–7 Hz)

The gateway to the subconscious

Theta waves are associated with deep relaxation, meditation, trance, and the border between sleep and wakefulness. This is often referred to as the "healing gateway" because it allows access to stored memories, symbolic imagery, and emotional patterns.

Associated with:

Hypnosis and guided imagery

Emotional memory processing

Enhanced creativity and intuition

Subconscious belief reprogramming

Access to trauma imprints and symbolic resolution

Theta is the frequency most often targeted in hypnotherapy and reprogramming techniques. In this state, the brain is receptive to new suggestions, making it ideal for rewriting emotional responses, releasing old patterns, and installing new neural pathways.

Alpha Waves (8–12 Hz)

The calm, restorative focus state

Alpha waves represent a state of relaxed alertness—neither fully focused nor deeply meditative. It's the classic "flow state," present during gentle focus, mindfulness, or quiet creativity.

Associated with:

Inner calm and emotional balance

Enhanced memory consolidation

Stress reduction

Integration of body and mind

Light trance and visualization

Alpha waves help bridge conscious and subconscious awareness, allowing a person to remain present while accessing deeper emotional content. Many meditative and breath-based practices aim to enhance alpha, as it's ideal for calming the nervous system while remaining mentally clear.

Beta Waves (13–30 Hz)

The thinking and action state

Beta waves dominate during active thinking, concentration, and problem solving. They're essential for navigating daily life, making decisions, and engaging with the external world.

Associated with:

Focus, planning, and analytical thinking

Verbal communication and mental effort

Logical problem-solving

Active attention

While necessary for productivity, excessive beta activity—especially in the higher ranges—can lead to anxiety, overthinking, and insomnia. This is the state most people operate in during stress or multitasking.

Healing typically requires a shift **out** of beta and into slower, more integrative frequencies like alpha, theta, and delta. However, some low-beta or SMR (sensorimotor rhythm) training has been used therapeutically to help with focus and neuroregulation in ADHD and sleep disorders.

Gamma Waves (30–100 Hz and beyond)

The integration and insight frequency

Gamma waves are the fastest brainwave frequency and are often associated with:

Moments of insight or peak consciousness

High-level cognitive functioning

Compassion and spiritual connection

Deep synchrony across different brain regions

Gamma activity has been observed in advanced meditators, such as Tibetan monks, during states of deep compassion and non-dual awareness. Gamma appears to support whole-brain coherence, integrating sensory, emotional, and cognitive experiences into unified insight.

In healing work, gamma may play a role after emotional integration has occurred, helping the brain solidify new patterns and gain expanded awareness.

Why brainwave balance matters in healing

Each brainwave state plays a distinct role. Healing and transformation occur not by suppressing one and enhancing another blindly, but by creating flexibility—the ability to move between states as needed.

For example:

Delta is essential for body repair

Theta allows access to subconscious programs

Alpha brings calm focus for integration

Beta enables action and cognitive clarity

Gamma supports insight and whole-brain resonance

When a person is stuck in one dominant state, especially high beta (chronic stress), the system becomes rigid. Healing becomes difficult. But when the brain can fluidly shift into slower, restorative frequencies, regeneration becomes possible.

This is why techniques like:

Hypnosis

Meditation

Brainwave entrainment

Breathwork

Sound therapy

...are powerful—they create the inner conditions where neuroplasticity, integration, and biological healing can occur.

Healing isn't just about calming the mind—It's about tuning the brain to the right frequency for transformation.

Binaural beats, isochronic tones, and sound entrainment

Tuning the brain into healing states with rhythmic stimuli.

In recent years, sound-based healing tools have gained increasing scientific credibility. Among them, binaural beats, isochronic tones, and sound entrainment stand out as non-invasive, low-cost methods for accessing altered states of consciousness—especially those associated with relaxation, neuroplasticity, and self-repair.

These auditory tools are based on a principle known as brainwave entrainment, the process by which rhythmic external stimuli cause the brain to align its natural frequency with the rhythm it is exposed to. When used purposefully, this creates a shortcut into desired states of consciousness—such as deep focus (alpha), subconscious access (theta), or physical repair (delta).

Let's explore how each of these tools works, what makes them different, and how they can be applied for therapeutic benefit.

Binaural beats: Creating a third frequency in the brain

Binaural beats work by playing two slightly different frequencies into each ear. For example:

Left ear: 200 Hz

Right ear: 210 Hz

The brain perceives a third tone: 10 Hz, which corresponds to alpha brainwave activity.

The ears do not hear this third tone in the air; instead, it is generated within the brainstem as a result of the two incoming signals. This phenomenon—called interaural phase difference—stimulates specific brainwave frequencies associated with relaxation, focus, meditation, or sleep.

Benefits of binaural beats (based on research):

Reduced anxiety and improved stress resilience

Enhanced memory and cognitive performance

Improved sleep and deep relaxation

Easier access to meditative and hypnotic states

Binaural beats require headphones to work properly, since the signal depends on separate input to each ear. The best results occur when listening in a quiet, distraction-free environment for at least 15–30 minutes.

Isochronic tones: Pulses of sound for stronger entrainment

Isochronic tones are single tones turned on and off rapidly at specific intervals—like a metronome for the brain. Unlike binaural beats, they do not require headphones, because the rhythmic pulsing is delivered to both ears simultaneously and directly entrains the brain.

Each tone is spaced to reflect a specific frequency. For example:

A tone pulsing 6 times per second (6 Hz) targets theta brainwave activity.

Because of their sharp, consistent rhythm, isochronic tones are often stronger and more immediately effective than binaural beats for some people—especially those who are neurodivergent, have difficulty meditating, or are new to sound-based practices.

Documented benefits:

Faster brainwave synchronization

Improved sleep onset

Better control over anxiety and intrusive thoughts

Enhanced focus and emotional regulation

Isochronic tones can be used with or without background music and are often embedded into guided meditations or therapeutic soundscapes.

Sound entrainment: Synchronizing the brain and body

Sound entrainment is the broader process of using any consistent rhythmic stimulus—sound, light, vibration, or movement—to synchronize the brain's activity with a desired frequency. It's not limited to artificial tones; it includes:

Drumming (used in indigenous cultures for altered states)

Chanting or toning (OM, mantras)

Rhythmic breathing or movement

Singing bowls, gongs, and tuning forks

Pulsed electromagnetic fields (PEMF) and vibroacoustic therapies

When used skillfully, sound entrainment can help regulate:

Heart rate variability (HRV)

Breath rhythm

Vagal tone (a key component of parasympathetic healing)

Limbic system activity (emotional regulation)

Motor synchronization (useful in trauma therapy and neurorehabilitation)

Over time, sound entrainment can train the brain to more easily access states of calm, safety, creativity, or sleep without external support—helping restore autonomic balance and improve self-regulation capacity.

Healing applications

Sound entrainment tools are now being incorporated into:

PTSD treatment protocols

Pain management programs

Fertility and stress reduction therapies

ADHD and learning support interventions

Deep relaxation and trauma processing practices

When paired with guided imagery, hypnosis, or neuroplastic practices, they amplify the therapeutic effect—by putting the brain in the exact state needed for memory reconsolidation, emotional processing, and somatic integration.

Sound is not just heard—it is felt, processed, and encoded. The brain doesn't just respond to words or logic. It responds to rhythm, tone, and pattern.

By learning to work with sound—not just as art, but as medicine—we unlock an ancient, science-backed key to healing from within.

Frequency medicine and its synergistic role in neuroregeneration

Bridging vibrational biology with brain repair

In recent years, a growing body of research has revealed something both profound and ancient: frequency affects biology. Every tissue, organ, and system in the body emits and responds to vibration—not just metaphorically, but electrically, electromagnetically, and acoustically. This understanding has given rise to a field often referred to as frequency medicine: a set of therapeutic approaches that use sound, light, electromagnetic fields, and vibrational resonance to influence cellular function, nervous system regulation, and tissue repair.

When applied with precision and intention, frequency medicine becomes a powerful adjunct to neuroregeneration. It doesn't replace biochemical or neurological treatments—it enhances them, by preparing the nervous system to shift out of chronic dysregulation and into a state where repair is possible.

The science of frequency and cellular response

At a fundamental level, all living cells are electrical entities. They communicate through ionic gradients, electromagnetic fields, and resonance. Cells "listen" to their environment through:

Membrane voltage (which regulates nutrient and signal exchange).

Mechanosensitive ion channels (which respond to sound and vibration).

Mitochondrial oscillation (which affects energy output and oxidative stress).

DNA transcription (which can be influenced by electromagnetic stimulation).

Disruption in the body's frequency field—whether from trauma, chronic stress, environmental toxins, or emotional dysregulation—can lead to biological incoherence: inflammation, nervous system rigidity, and poor cellular communication.

Conversely, exposure to harmonic frequencies (through sound, light, or pulsed electromagnetic fields) has been shown to:

Increase cellular ATP production (mitochondrial support)

Modulate calcium signaling and neural excitability

Stimulate neurotrophic factors like BDNF (Brain-Derived Neurotrophic Factor)

Enhance synaptic repair and neuroplasticity

Reduce inflammatory cytokines and oxidative stress

The nervous system as a frequency processor

The brain is exquisitely responsive to frequency. In fact, it operates through frequency—its states of consciousness are measurable in brainwave patterns (delta, theta, alpha, beta, gamma), which correspond to attention, relaxation, creativity, and repair. The autonomic nervous system, too, responds to rhythmic stimuli: heartbeats, breath cycles, circadian rhythms, and sensory input.

When these rhythms become disorganized—due to unresolved trauma, chronic overstimulation, or disconnection from natural cycles—healing slows or halts. This is why re-establishing coherent frequencies through therapeutic means can restore the brain's ability to:

Transition between states smoothly (neuroflexibility)

Regulate pain and inflammation

Access deeper states of rest, integration, and learning

Engage the parasympathetic nervous system (rest-and-repair mode)

Modalities of frequency medicine supporting neuroregeneration

Several therapeutic tools are being studied and clinically applied in the realm of frequency-based neurorepair:

1. Pulsed Electromagnetic Field Therapy (PEMF)

Low-frequency EM pulses stimulate cellular voltage and bone/tissue repair.

Used in neurological rehab to improve circulation, reduce inflammation, and support myelination.

2. Low-Level Laser Therapy (LLLT / Photobiomodulation).

Infrared and red light influence mitochondrial function and gene expression.

Has shown promise in treating traumatic brain injury, neurodegeneration, and inflammation.

3. Sound Therapy (Binaural Beats, Singing Bowls, Voice Toning).

Stimulates brainwave entrainment, emotional integration, and vagal tone

Supports mental clarity, emotional regulation, and subconscious access.

4. Biofield and Vibrational Therapies (Tuning forks, Somatic vibration).

Noninvasive methods that reintroduce rhythmic coherence to the body's subtle fields.

Used to resolve emotional imprints, trauma loops, and energetic stagnation.

These modalities do not act in isolation. When paired with hypnosis, neuroplasticity work, and intentional lifestyle changes, they create a synergistic effect: each layer reinforcing the others, amplifying the nervous system's capacity to reorganize and heal.

Why frequency must be part of the regeneration conversation?

Regeneration is not only cellular—it is systemic and informational. The body cannot regenerate while locked in defensive patterns. Frequency medicine helps unlock those patterns, bringing coherence where there was chaos, flow where there was stagnation.

When frequency therapy is used as part of an integrative approach to brain healing:

The brain becomes more plastic

The mind becomes more receptive

The body becomes more cooperative

The healing becomes more profound

Frequency is not just a healing tool—It is the language of the body.

When we learn to speak it, we stop forcing healing... and start resonating with it.

Hypnosis as an entrainment tool to access optimal brain states

Guiding the brain into regeneration through rhythmic suggestion and focused awareness

Hypnosis is often misunderstood as a form of sleep or mind control. In reality, it is a natural, trainable state of focused attention and neurophysiological alignment—one that allows the brain to enter optimal frequencies for healing, learning, and regeneration.

What makes hypnosis so effective is not just its psychological effect—it is its ability to entrain the brain into highly specific states of consciousness, particularly within the alpha, theta, and delta brainwave ranges. These states are not only more relaxed—they are neurologically suited to change.

In this sense, hypnosis is not just a therapeutic technique.It is a form of neural entrainment—a guided recalibration of brain function.

Hypnosis and brainwave shifts

The act of entering a hypnotic trance—through breath, suggestion, and focused imagery—produces measurable changes in brainwave activity:

From high beta (alert, stressed thinking) →

To alpha (calm focus) →

To theta (subconscious access) →

Sometimes into delta (deep repair and unconscious processing).

These transitions are not incidental—they are the goal of hypnosis. When the brain shifts into these frequencies, the following occurs:

The critical factor of the conscious mind relaxes.

Subconscious material becomes accessible.

Plasticity-enhancing chemicals (like acetylcholine and serotonin) increase.

The autonomic nervous system rebalances, favoring parasympathetic dominance (rest and repair).

The client becomes more open to new associations, beliefs, and sensory integration.

These are the very conditions required for lasting therapeutic change—especially when it involves rewiring emotional patterns, breaking trauma loops, or promoting somatic healing.

Entrainment through voice, rhythm, and repetition

Hypnosis works because it follows the principles of entrainment—the brain's natural tendency to synchronize with external rhythmic input. In this case, the "input" is:

The hypnotist's voice cadence

Paced breathing and progressive relaxation

Repetitive suggestion patterns

Rhythmic imagery or metaphors

Embedded commands timed to the client's breath or eye movement

As the session deepens, these rhythmic cues gently guide the brain into its target state. Unlike external technologies like binaural beats or pulsed light, hypnosis uses internal rhythm and meaning as the primary entrainment tool. This is why its effects can be more profound and enduring—it builds resonance through relationship and language.

Why these states are ideal for healing

The brain states most commonly accessed in hypnosis (especially theta and alpha) are associated with:

Enhanced emotional processing.

Decreased amygdala reactivity (less fear and hypervigilance).

Increased access to stored memory and belief structures.

Heightened imagination, creativity, and problem solving.

Improved connectivity between brain hemispheres and networks (such as the DMN and salience network).

These neurological conditions are ideal for reprogramming dysfunctional patterns that maintain physical symptoms, emotional reactivity, or psychological resistance to change.

In deeper trance, delta waves may emerge—supporting tissue repair, hormonal reset, immune modulation, and unconscious integration. When paired with positive suggestion and somatic imagery, this state supports regenerative healing, not just psychological insight.

Hypnosis as a gateway, not just a tool

In the context of neuroregeneration, hypnosis is far more than a tool for suggestion—it becomes a gateway into an optimal neural environment. Once this state is reached, the mind becomes more receptive to:

Self-directed healing

Lifestyle changes

Integration of frequency therapy

Emotional reframing

Memory reconsolidation

Cellular repair processes triggered by rest-and-repair physiology

This is one reason why integrative approaches like HypnoCell® include brainwave entrainment through hypnosis as the foundation for deeper interventions—because nothing takes root in the nervous system without access to the proper state.

Healing isn't just about what we say to the mind—It's about when and how we say it.

Hypnosis creates the inner rhythm for healing to land, unfold, and regenerate.

Chapter 5

Hypnosis as a pathway to regeneration

In the search for regeneration—whether of cells, tissue, immunity, or emotional resilience—medicine has often focused on external solutions: drugs, surgeries, supplements, or physical interventions. But one of the most powerful tools for activating healing doesn't come from outside the body—it comes from within the brain itself.

Hypnosis is not a mystical or fringe practice. It is a clinically recognized state of focused attention and altered consciousness that creates a neurobiological environment ideal for healing. It is a doorway to the subconscious and unconscious mind, where many of the patterns that shape our health are stored and maintained. More importantly, hypnosis can serve as a pathway to regeneration—not just mental, but physiological, when used with precision and purpose.

Through carefully guided hypnosis, the nervous system is invited to shift from defense to repair, from stress to safety, from disconnection to coherence. In this state, the body becomes more receptive to healing because the mind finally stops resisting it.

What makes hypnosis regenerative?

Healing requires more than desire—it requires access. Many people intellectually want to feel better, but their deeper mind remains in a state of alarm, holding onto patterns of fear, tension, or protective suppression. Hypnosis works because it bypasses the critical mind, the gatekeeper of resistance, and creates a direct pathway to the subconscious and unconscious systems that control:

Immune modulation

Hormonal balance

Pain perception

Stress responses

Regeneration and tissue repair

Beliefs, memories, and meaning

By guiding the brain into slow-wave states like alpha, theta, and delta, hypnosis activates the very same pathways involved in neuroplasticity and cellular renewal. This is where the true work of healing begins—not by forcing the body to comply, but by retraining the mind to allow it.

The science of hypnotic regeneration

Numerous studies using EEG and fMRI have shown that hypnosis alters brain activity in regions critical to healing:

The anterior cingulate cortex, which governs emotional pain and internal conflict.

The insula, which regulates interoception and body awareness.

The amygdala, where fear and trauma loops are encoded.

The default mode network, responsible for self-perception and internal narrative.

The autonomic nervous system, which controls stress vs. rest-and-repair modes.

In the hypnotic state, the brain shows increased neuroplasticity, reduced threat perception, and greater integration between cognitive and emotional centers. This paves the way for a cascade of healing responses:

Lower cortisol and systemic inflammation

Improved immune signaling

Normalization of hormonal rhythms

Relaxation of chronic muscular tension

Activation of regenerative processes in tissue, gut, and skin

Enhanced openness to behavioral and lifestyle change

Repatterning the healing loop

Hypnosis doesn't just create a moment of relaxation—it allows the brain to revisit and rewire stored imprints that have kept the body locked in illness, dysfunction, or pain. These imprints may include:

Traumatic memories

Limiting subconscious beliefs

Suppressed emotions

Somatic memories stored in tissues

Repetitive stress patterns encoded into the nervous system

Once these patterns are accessed in a safe, trance-induced state, they can be:

Reframed with more adaptive meaning.

Released through visualization, somatic awareness, or symbolic completion.

Rewritten with new internal instructions for safety, vitality, and cellular coherence.

This is why hypnosis can be so effective in chronic conditions that have resisted conventional approaches—not because it magically removes disease, but because it resolves the internal conditions that have prevented healing from occurring.

From stress physiology to regenerative potential

Most people live in a chronic state of sympathetic dominance—what we call "fight or flight." In this state, the body:

Diverts resources away from digestion, fertility, and immunity

Suppresses repair hormones and growth factors

Produces inflammatory cytokines

Remains primed for threat detection, not restoration

Hypnosis creates the opposite: a shift into parasympathetic dominance, also known as "rest and repair" mode. Here, the nervous system cues:

Tissue repair and wound healing

Hormonal recalibration

Emotional integration

Vagal tone activation

Rebalancing of the gut-brain axis

In this state, regeneration is no longer resisted—it's allowed.

Hypnosis within a regenerative protocol

When used within a comprehensive healing system—such as HypnoCell®—hypnosis becomes more than relaxation. It becomes:

A priming mechanism for frequency-based therapies (like sound or PEMF).

A delivery system for subconscious reprogramming.

A reset button for autonomic imbalance.

A bridge between biology and belief, between intention and integration.

It allows the individual to step out of survival mode and into biological coherence, creating conditions that no supplement or medication can produce on its own.

Regeneration is not something you force.

It's something your body knows how to do—Once your brain is entrained to allow it.

How therapeutic hypnosis differs from entertainment myths

Separating clinical reality from stage fiction

When people hear the word hypnosis, they often picture a swinging pocket watch, a dramatic countdown, or a stage performer making someone cluck like a chicken. These theatrical portrayals—while amusing—have contributed to decades of misunderstanding and stigma around a therapeutic method that is both powerful and evidence-based.

In truth, clinical hypnosis bears little resemblance to stage hypnosis. One is designed for spectacle and illusion; the other is structured for precision, healing, and deep psychological and physiological transformation.

Clinical hypnosis: The therapeutic model

Therapeutic hypnosis is a collaborative and voluntary process that uses verbal guidance and focused attention to help a person enter a specific brain state—one that facilitates:

Access to subconscious patterns and stored emotional material

Enhanced neuroplasticity and responsiveness to suggestion

Decreased activity in the brain's default mode network (overthinking and self-criticism)

Regulation of the autonomic nervous system (stress vs. healing)

The practitioner's role is not to "control" the subject but to create safety, focus, and a state of internal readiness where healing can unfold from within.

In clinical settings, hypnosis is used to:

Alleviate chronic pain

Support trauma resolution

Improve immune and hormonal regulation

Manage anxiety and phobias

Accelerate recovery from illness or surgery

Access and resolve subconscious roots of chronic conditions

In systems like HypnoCell®, hypnosis also helps establish the ideal neurophysiological state for regeneration, particularly when combined with frequency-based therapies and lifestyle integration.

Stage hypnosis: Entertainment, not therapy

By contrast, stage hypnosis is designed to entertain, often relying on:

Group dynamics and peer pressure

Rapid inductions in highly suggestible individuals

Pre-screened volunteers

Exaggerated behaviors to amuse an audience

These performances use hypnosis—but they use it superficially and often reinforce the myth that hypnosis is about:

Loss of control

Mindless obedience

Embarrassing acts

Vulnerability or unconsciousness

In truth, no one can be hypnotized against their will, and even in deep trance, individuals maintain full awareness of their values, limits, and surroundings.

The Core Differences at a Glance:

Why the difference matters

These myths aren't just harmless—they prevent people from seeking help. Many who could benefit from therapeutic hypnosis hesitate because they fear:

Being manipulated

Losing control

Being embarrassed

"Getting stuck" in trance

Remembering painful material

But therapeutic hypnosis is none of those things. In fact, it is empowering, client-directed, and neurologically safe. In trained hands, hypnosis becomes a bridge between awareness and biology—offering a way to access change that is often inaccessible through willpower or conscious reasoning alone.

In the HypnoCell® model, hypnosis is not just a technique—it is the entry point into a state of neurological coherence, where real regeneration begins.

Hypnosis doesn't take away control.

It helps you reclaim it—from the inside out.

Accessing regenerative states through deep trance

Why depth of consciousness matters for healing and rewiring

Healing is not just a physical event—it is also a neurological and energetic recalibration. While medicine tends to focus on biochemical pathways, true and lasting regeneration often depends on accessing the deeper layers of the nervous system—those beneath conscious control. This is where trance becomes not only helpful but essential.

Deep trance, a therapeutic state accessed through clinical hypnosis, is a form of altered consciousness in which the brain shifts into slower wave frequencies (theta and delta), enabling access to internal systems that regulate emotion, immune response, memory, and repair. It is not unconsciousness, nor is it sleep—it is a highly focused, internally directed state of awareness that allows the body to enter the most receptive conditions for healing.

What happens in deep trance?

When someone enters a deep hypnotic trance, several important things occur neurologically and physiologically:

The default mode network (DMN)—responsible for self-referential thought and inner chatter—quietly disengages. This creates space for new connections and meanings to emerge.

Brainwave activity slows, usually into the theta range (4–8 Hz) or even delta (0.5–4 Hz). These frequencies are associated with deep integration, emotional resolution, and physical regeneration.

Neurochemical changes occur, including increases in serotonin, oxytocin, and brain-derived neurotrophic factor (BDNF)—substances associated with neuroplasticity, safety, and healing.

The autonomic nervous system shifts from sympathetic (fight-or-flight) to parasympathetic dominance (rest-and-repair), activating physiological repair mechanisms throughout the body.

In this state, the conscious mind steps back, allowing access to the subconscious and unconscious regions where emotional imprints, trauma loops, and autonomic conditioning reside. This is critical, because most chronic issues—whether physical, emotional, or behavioral—are maintained by subconscious programs that are resistant to willpower alone.

Trance as a biological healing environment

Deep trance doesn't heal in and of itself—it simply creates the internal conditions for healing to become possible again. Just as surgery requires a sterile field and proper anesthesia, regeneration requires:

Safety

Stillness

Receptivity

Neurochemical support

Mental and emotional alignment

Trance provides all of these. It acts as a regenerative ecosystem, giving the brain permission to:

Release hypervigilance and unresolved memories

Process unintegrated emotions stored in the body

Rewrite internal narratives that affect hormonal and immune balance

Reconnect disconnected neural networks

Send coherent instructions to cells, tissues, and systems

Why depth matters

While light trance is useful for habit change or stress reduction, deep trance is often required for foundational reprogramming and neuroregeneration. In this depth:

The body is more responsive to guided imagery, frequency therapy, and vibrational inputs.

Longstanding emotional blocks can be accessed without resistance.

The subconscious is more impressionable—making suggestions for healing more effective.

Somatic memory (stored in tissues) becomes more available for release and integration.

This is the level of trance we intentionally activate in the HypnoCell® method—because the body cannot fully regenerate if the brain is still defending itself.

To heal deeply, the body must first feel safe.

Deep trance is the state where safety, surrender, and cellular repair meet.

Case studies: Chronic pain, trauma recovery, and immune modulation

How hypnotic states support healing in real-world clinical scenarios

To understand the impact of hypnosis in regenerative medicine, it helps to look beyond theory and into the lived experience of healing. The following clinical case studies illustrate how deep hypnotic work—combined with neuroplastic insights and frequency-based entrainment—can support profound shifts in physical symptoms, emotional resilience, and biological regulation.

Each case highlights a different physiological domain, yet shares a common thread: traditional interventions had reached a plateau. It was only through accessing subconscious patterns, somatic imprints, and regenerative brain states that lasting change occurred.

Case 1: Chronic pain and the nervous system "loop"

Patient: 47-year-old woman with fibromyalgia and persistent lower back pain.

History: 12 years of pain, unresponsive to physiotherapy, painkillers, and lifestyle changes.

Approach: After identifying early emotional trauma stored in the body, the patient was guided through a series of trance-based sessions focusing on:

Neural re-patterning of pain perception (via metaphor and imagery),

Accessing the pain memory at the subconscious level,

Reframing the body's pain signal from "threat" to "attention request",

Embedding new safety cues into the nervous system.

Result: After 6 sessions over 10 weeks, the patient reported:

60% reduction in baseline pain,

Improved sleep and digestion,

Decreased dependency on medication,

The ability to differentiate between emotional stress pain and true physiological strain.

Clinical insight:

Pain is not always a direct measure of tissue damage—it is often a neural prediction rooted in unresolved emotion, memory, or defense physiology. Hypnosis helps rewrite this prediction.

Case 2: Trauma recovery and nervous system coherence

Patient: 33-year-old male, survivor of a car accident with PTSD and panic attacks.

History: Nightmares, hypervigilance, intrusive images, and digestive issues.

Approach: The hypnosis protocol focused on:

Establishing physiological safety through breath entrainment and somatic anchoring,

Accessing the trauma memory in trance without re-traumatization,

Re-integrating sensory fragments into a coherent narrative,

Guided visualization of post-trauma identity reconstruction.

Result: Within 8 weeks:

Panic episodes ceased

Nighttime sleep extended from 3 to 7 hours

Significant emotional stability, reduced startle response

Gradual return to work and social life

Clinical insight:

Trauma is not stored as a story—it's stored **as** disruption in sensory and emotional coherence. Hypnosis re-links these fragments under conditions of internal safety.

Case 3: Immune dysregulation and autoimmunity

Patient: 41-year-old woman with Hashimoto's thyroiditis.

History: Fluctuating TSH levels, fatigue, hair loss, and emotional overwhelm. Conventional treatment plateaued.

Approach: Integrative hypnosis sessions addressed:

Subconscious identity conflicts around self-protection and control,

Emotional resonance of chronic overgiving and "attack from within",

Regulation of autonomic states (calming sympathetic dominance),

Visualization of immune cells restoring balance and discernment.

Result: Within 12 weeks:

Improved energy levels and mood

TSH stabilized (confirmed by endocrinologist)

Hair regrowth and improved digestion

Reduction in perceived stress and reactivity to food triggers

Clinical insight:

The immune system responds to more than antigens—it responds to perception, belief, and stress physiology. Hypnosis helps rewire the narrative that informs immune behavior.

Common threads across all cases

While the specific symptoms varied, these case studies share key themes:

Conventional treatments alone were insufficient.

Patients felt "stuck" in loops their minds could not explain.

Healing began once the subconscious language of the body was addressed.

Trance allowed safe exploration of emotional material without re-traumatization.

The brain's natural plasticity was activated through deep inner alignment.

Frequency, meaning, and focused suggestion accelerated neurobiological change.

Healing is not about erasing symptoms.

It's about reclaiming the internal conditions in which health can re-emerge.

Chapter 6

Neural recalibration

The human brain is not a passive recorder of experience—it is an active prediction machine. Every thought, sensation, and response is filtered through an internal model shaped by past experiences, emotional associations, and perceived threats. When this model becomes distorted—through trauma, chronic stress, or unresolved emotional memory—the brain begins to generate inaccurate predictions about the body and the world. These predictions influence everything from immune response and hormonal output to pain perception and emotional reactivity.

Neural recalibration is the process of resetting these faulty predictive patterns and bringing the nervous system back into alignment with the present moment. It is not about erasing the past, but updating the brain's operating system—teaching it that safety, vitality, and possibility are now available.

How neural patterns become mismatched

When the brain detects danger—real or perceived—it encodes that experience through:

Increased amygdala activity (fear and vigilance)

Autonomic imprinting (fight, flight, freeze, or fawn)

Subconscious conclusions ("I'm not safe", "My body is failing", "I'm not allowed to rest")

Somatic memory held in muscle tension, breathing, and organ function

Over time, these responses become default programs, even when the original threat is gone. This leads to:

Chronic inflammation

Pain without injury

Hormonal imbalance

Autoimmune activation

Emotional shutdown or hyperreactivity

The inability to relax, digest, or regenerate

The brain is not doing this maliciously—it's simply repeating a pattern it believes is protective.

Recalibrating the predictive brain

Neural recalibration involves disrupting maladaptive patterns and establishing new neurological associations based on safety, coherence, and integration.

This process requires:

Accessing the subconscious (where old beliefs and emotional scripts are stored)

Entering neuroplastic states (alpha, theta, or delta brainwaves)

Providing alternative sensory and emotional inputs (e.g., guided imagery, somatic safety cues)

Reinforcing new patterns through repetition and emotional resonance

Techniques like hypnosis, neurofeedback, EMDR, and frequency entrainment are especially effective because they bypass conscious resistance and allow bottom-up reprogramming of the nervous system.

The role of hypnosis in neural recalibration

Hypnosis facilitates neural recalibration by:

Quieting the analytical mind

Creating space for new associations

Allowing emotional memory to surface in a safe, guided way

Embedding new narratives and imagery that the brain begins to accept as truth

Guiding the body into rest-and-repair physiology, where change is biologically supported

In models like HypnoCell®, neural recalibration is central to the healing process. We do not try to suppress symptoms, but rather teach the brain to stop misinterpreting them as threats. This shifts the entire healing loop—from chronic defense to regenerative coherence.

Signs of successful neural recalibration

When the brain begins to shift, clients often report:

Sudden relief of long-held tension

Emotional release without re-traumatization

Improved sleep and digestion

A new sense of "neutrality" around past memories

Decreased symptom intensity, even without medical changes

Spontaneous insights and behavioral shifts

These are not coincidences—they are signs that the brain has updated its model, and the body is no longer trapped in a loop of outdated responses.

Healing doesn't always require new tools.

Sometimes it requires a new instruction set—One that the nervous system can finally believe.

The Hypnocell® model: Entering trance, identifying the signal, creating the reframe

The HypnoCell® method was developed to bridge neuroscience, regenerative medicine, and therapeutic hypnosis into a practical, repeatable process for activating healing. It is grounded in the understanding that chronic symptoms are not random—they are informational signals from the nervous system, shaped by past experiences and internal perceptions.

In this model, symptoms are seen not as malfunctions to suppress, but as encoded messages from the subconscious and unconscious mind—messages that can be translated, recontextualized, and updated once the brain is in the right state.

The HypnoCell® framework moves through three essential phases:

Entering Trance

Identifying the Signal

Creating the Reframe

Each step is crucial to initiating true neurological recalibration and systemic regeneration.

1. Entering trance: Accessing the neuroplastic state

The process begins by guiding the individual into a safe, focused, and altered state of consciousness—commonly referred to as trance. This is not sleep or loss of control. It is a neurologically distinct state marked by:

Reduced cortical resistance

Slower brainwaves (theta or alpha)

Increased suggestibility and imagination

Parasympathetic dominance (rest, repair, digestion)

In this state, the conscious mind softens, allowing therapeutic access to deeper layers of memory, belief, and somatic experience.

Techniques used to enter trance may include:

Guided breath and body awareness

Progressive relaxation or somatic anchoring

Rhythmic language patterns

Visualization and metaphor

Frequency entrainment (binaural beats, delta-theta tones)

This step prepares the nervous system to update long-held scripts and shift out of survival-based neural loops.

2. Identifying the signal: Tracing the origin of the pattern

Once in trance, the client is gently guided to locate the "neural signal"—the subconscious pattern or emotional imprint underlying the symptom. This may be:

An unresolved emotional event (often preverbal or symbolic)

A limiting belief ("I am not safe," "Healing isn't possible")

A body memory or somatic echo (tightness, heat, numbness, etc.)

A protective strategy (avoidance, shutdown, hypervigilance)

The signal is not always logical or linear. The subconscious often stores information as:

Images

Sensory fragments

Symbols

Felt experiences in the body

Through gentle questioning, regression (if needed), or metaphor, the practitioner helps bring the root mismatch into awareness—not to relive it, but to witness and decode it safely.

The act of locating the signal is in itself reparative. It tells the brain: "You are safe enough now to process this."

3. Creating the reframe: Delivering new instructions to the nervous system.

Once the original imprint or faulty perception is revealed, the next phase is to reframe it.

This does not mean denying reality or replacing pain with false positivity. Instead, it means:

Introducing a new, adaptive interpretation of the experience

Embedding safety, agency, and permission into the neural narrative

Offering the body a corrective experience in real time

Reassociating the symptom with resolution rather than threat

Examples of reframes might include:

"What happened to me does not define my future."

"My body can remember safety."

"The pain was protecting me. I can now release it."

"I am no longer in that environment. I am here now."

This is where neural recalibration begins: the brain receives updated information, and the body responds. The individual may feel a release of tension, tears, warmth, or even spontaneous insight. These are not coincidences—they are signs of integration.

Repetition, integration, and lifestyle support

The HypnoCell® process is not a one-time reset. After the reframe, ongoing support helps the brain reinforce the new neural pathway. This is achieved through:

Self-hypnosis practices

Journaling and embodiment exercises

Regenerative breathwork or movement

Environmental reinforcement (daily cues of safety and alignment)

Nutritional and lifestyle choices that support neuroplasticity

By combining subconscious rewiring with daily behavioral alignment, the HypnoCell® method stabilizes the shift—moving from momentary insight to lasting regeneration.

Symptoms are signals.

The brain is plastic.

And healing begins the moment you change the message.

Installing regenerative instructions in neuroplastic loops

How to guide the brain into repetition that repairs instead of protects

The human brain is a pattern-making organ. It encodes repeated experiences—both emotional and physical—into what we call neural loops: familiar, automatic circuits that determine how we think, feel, behave, and heal. These loops are essential for survival. They help us learn quickly, avoid danger, and conserve energy. But when they are based on outdated or distorted inputs—such as unresolved trauma, chronic stress, or inherited beliefs—they can block healing, create dysfunction, and reinforce the very states we seek to escape.

The good news is: these loops are plastic. They can be interrupted, redirected, and—most importantly—reprogrammed with new instructions for regeneration.

This is one of the foundational principles of the HypnoCell™ approach.

Neuroplastic loops: The engine of habit and healing

Neuroplasticity refers to the brain's ability to change its structure and function in response to experience. This is not limited to childhood—it continues throughout life. However, the brain does not distinguish between helpful **and** unhelpful patterns—it simply repeats what it knows.

Common examples of maladaptive loops include:

Chronic pain reinforced by protective tension

Fatigue cycles sustained by beliefs of unworthiness or danger

Immune suppression linked to unresolved grief or shame

Hypervigilance and cortisol spikes triggered by subconscious memory

These patterns feel automatic because they are. They've been rehearsed so many times that they've become the brain's default setting.

But with targeted hypnotic intervention and a precise delivery of new information, these loops can be rewritten.

What are "regenerative instructions"?

Regenerative instructions are therapeutic suggestions delivered during trance, specifically designed to:

Interrupt maladaptive neural firing patterns,

Install adaptive alternatives rooted in safety, coherence, and vitality,

Activate the body's innate repair systems, including immune, endocrine, and nervous responses,

Reinforce a future-oriented identity that aligns with healing,

These instructions can take the form of:

Symbolic imagery (e.g., "cells glowing with clarity and communication")

Embedded affirmations (e.g., "It is now safe to regenerate")

Somatic suggestions (e.g., "Your breath knows how to carry healing to every cell")

Visualized outcomes (e.g., "You feel light, calm, and whole as your body remembers wellness")

The precision of the language and the emotional tone of delivery are key. The brain learns best when:

It feels emotionally safe

It's in a receptive state (theta or alpha)

It is engaged in imagery and rhythm

The information feels true enough to try

The process of installation

Access the neuroplastic state:

Through trance, frequency entrainment, or meditative focus, the brain shifts into a mode where it's more willing to revise its patterns.

Disrupt the old loop:

The symptom or belief is named, acknowledged, and understood—not as a problem, but as a message or adaptation that is no longer needed.

Deliver the new instruction:

Through hypnotic suggestion, metaphor, or imagery, the nervous system is given an upgraded message: one that promotes regulation, rest, immune clarity, or growth.

Emotionally encode the new loop:

The more emotionally meaningful the instruction, the more quickly and deeply it takes hold. Emotion is the glue of memory.

Reinforce and rehearse:

With self-hypnosis, breathwork, journaling, and conscious behavior, the loop is strengthened and eventually becomes the new default.

Example: From protection loop to regeneration loop

Old Loop:

"I must stay on high alert to survive"→ Constant tension → Fatigue → Immune suppression → Chronic symptoms

Intervention:Through trance, the root belief is identified and honored. The body is guided into safety. New imagery and suggestion are introduced.

New Loop Installed:

"I am safe now. My body can shift from defense to repair."→ Calm vagal tone → Better digestion, rest, and immune modulation→ Reduction in chronic symptoms→ Brain associates safety with healing, not vigilance

Why It Works

This is not simply mental reprogramming—it's neurological entrainment.

The brain rewires itself in response to:

What it believes to be true

What it feels repeatedly

What it practices with presence

HypnoCell® uses this truth with care and precision: not to bypass medical interventions, but to support them by aligning the brain's instructions with the body's regenerative potential.

The body follows the brain.

The brain follows belief.

And belief can be re-authored—one loop at a time.

Reinforcement and subconscious "rehearsal"

How lasting change is built through repetition in the neuroplastic mind

One of the most important—and often overlooked—elements of healing is reinforcement. It's not enough to introduce new neural patterns or regenerative instructions once. For the brain to adopt and maintain change, it must rehearse these new patterns repeatedly until they become more familiar than the old ones.

This process is called subconscious rehearsal—a form of internal practice that occurs outside of conscious effort, and which drives neuroplasticity in ways that are both powerful and sustainable.

Why the brain needs repetition

The brain doesn't change because of insight alone.It changes because of consistency.

When a person experiences a new emotional truth, insight, or healing instruction during hypnosis or deep trance, it creates an opening—a window of plasticity in which new synaptic connections can form. But for those connections to strengthen and stabilize, they must be reinforced.

This is where subconscious rehearsal comes in: the repetition of an internal experience that the brain practices as if it were real.

Neuroscience shows that:

The brain cannot easily distinguish between real experience and vividly imagined experience.

Mental rehearsal activates the same neural pathways as actual behavior.

Repeating a visualization, sensation, or belief enhances myelination of the associated circuits, making the pattern stronger and more automatic.

In other words, what you rehearse internally becomes what you default to externally.

Subconscious rehearsal in action

After a HypnoCell® session, the subconscious has been given new material:

"It is safe to rest."

"My body can regenerate."

"I am no longer under threat."

"Healing is possible now."

But the subconscious operates on familiarity and survival, not logic. It requires evidence and repetition to replace old protective loops with new regenerative ones. This is where reinforcement becomes critical.

Rehearsal can take several forms:

Self-hypnosis recordings that repeat and deepen the healing instructions

Guided visualizations that replay the transformation experienced in trance

Daily rituals (breathing, movement, journaling) that anchor the new identity

Somatic cues that remind the nervous system of its new safety pattern (e.g., relaxed posture, grounding touch, scent, sound)

Each time the new belief or image is rehearsed, the brain updates its prediction model—and what was once "foreign" becomes "familiar."

Why old patterns try to return—and how rehearsal stops them

Old neural loops often feel stronger, not because they are "truer," but because they've been rehearsed longer. After a breakthrough, it's common for the brain to test the new pattern by revisiting the old one—especially under stress.

This isn't failure. It's just a system seeking reinforcement.

By consciously and subconsciously rehearsing the new state (even briefly), the brain gets the message:

"Yes, this is still the direction we're going."

Over time, the old loop weakens from lack of use. The new one strengthens through focused attention, emotional tone, and repetition.

Building reinforcement into daily life

The HypnoCell® model encourages reinforcement through:

Nighttime audio protocols that deepen the healing message in theta/delta brain states

Anchoring phrases repeated at key transition points in the day (waking, eating, resting)

Somatic reinforcement (e.g., gentle touch while saying: "I am safe now")

Environmental alignment: surrounding oneself with cues of the desired internal state (music, lighting, routines)

Healing becomes not just something that "happened in session," but something the body lives into, practices, and stabilizes.

The subconscious doesn't care if something is new or good.

It cares if it's familiar.

Make healing familiar—and it becomes your new baseline.

Emotional coherence and biological response

How aligning emotion, thought, and physiology unlocks regeneration

One of the most overlooked drivers of chronic illness and stalled healing is not purely physical — it is the lack of coherence between what we think, what we feel, and what our bodies believe to be true.

The emerging fields of psychoneuroimmunology and neurocardiology show us that emotional states do not merely influence biology—they shape it continuously, down to the level of gene expression, hormone output, and cellular repair.

When our emotions, thoughts, and bodily states are misaligned or conflicted, the body remains in a state of incoherence, often stuck in subtle or overt survival physiology. But when we achieve emotional coherence — when the heart, brain, and nervous system are aligned in a state of safety and openness — we see profound shifts in biological processes that support healing.

What is emotional coherence?

Emotional coherence is a state in which:

The emotions you feel,

The thoughts you think,

And the signals your body sendsare all congruent and working together.

For example, if someone consciously says, "I want to heal," but deep inside they feel terrified, undeserving, or braced for disappointment, the body detects the conflict and responds with protective physiology:

Increased cortisol

Muscle tension

Suppressed immune signaling

Shallow breathing

Defensive autonomic patterns

This is emotional incoherence, and it creates a subtle but powerful blockade against regeneration.

By contrast, when your emotions, beliefs, and body cues are aligned — when your entire system genuinely feels and believes "I am safe, it is possible to heal, I can allow restoration now" — your biology shifts into a state optimized for:

Cellular repair

Immune recalibration

Hormonal balance

Digestive restoration

Neurological plasticity

How coherence drives biological change

Research by institutions like the HeartMath Institute has demonstrated that coherent emotional states (e.g., appreciation, calm, compassion) produce smoother heart rate variability (HRV) patterns, which in turn send regulating signals to the brain and other organs. This heart-brain synchronization influences:

Reduced amygdala overactivity (less fear and hypervigilance),

Increased vagal tone (improved parasympathetic dominance),

Balanced hypothalamic-pituitary-adrenal (HPA) axis function (better stress resilience),

Enhanced production of regenerative hormones like DHEA and growth factors.

Meanwhile, positive emotional states have been shown to:

Lower inflammatory cytokines

Increase secretory IgA (frontline immune defense)

Support mitochondrial efficiency (better cellular energy)

This means that emotional coherence is not just a "nice feeling"—it is a measurable biological event that changes how your body repairs and protects itself.

Emotional incoherence: The invisible block to healing

Many people with chronic conditions unknowingly live in a state of emotional conflict.

They consciously want health, but subconsciously carry fear, guilt, or an identity tied to being unwell.

They try to think positively, but their bodies remain tense, breath shallow, heart rhythms erratic.

They pursue treatments, but internally anticipate failure or abandonment.

This lack of coherence sends mixed signals to the nervous system, which prioritizes protection over regeneration.The result? Healing slows, symptoms persist, and the body stays locked in outdated patterns.

The body does not simply respond to treatments.It responds to the internal environment of belief and emotion.

When you create coherence, you unlock a biology that wants to heal.

······•··•·•···

Chapter 7
Lifestyle as neural input

When people think of "lifestyle," they often think of nutrition, exercise, or sleep purely in metabolic or cardiovascular terms. But lifestyle is far more than a series of health boxes to check—it is a continuous stream of input that shapes the brain, rewires the nervous system, and directly instructs the body on how to function.

Your brain is not a sealed computer that simply runs on inherited software. It is dynamic, impressionable, and constantly updating itself based on the signals it receives. Every thought, every breath, every bite of food, every social interaction, and every hour of sleep or stress becomes data your nervous system uses to decide:

How safe you are

How to allocate resources (toward repair or defense)

Which genes to express

Whether to prioritize growth, immunity, digestion, and fertility—or to keep the system in survival mode.

In this sense, lifestyle is neural input. It is not just about physical health. It literally sculpts your brain's wiring, your emotional regulation, and your body's capacity to regenerate.

How lifestyle acts as continuous programming

Every choice and habit you maintain sends repetitive messages to your nervous system and shapes your neurobiology:

Nutrition as an informational signal

Nutrients are not just fuel; they are molecular instructions. Omega-3s, polyphenols, B vitamins, and amino acids modulate neurotransmitter production, reduce neuroinflammation, and support synaptic plasticity. Meanwhile, chronic intake of processed foods and excess sugars can drive oxidative stress, glycation, and microglial priming—keeping the brain in a pro-inflammatory state.

Sleep as neural recalibration

During deep sleep (especially slow-wave sleep), the brain performs critical housekeeping: consolidating memories, pruning unnecessary synapses, and flushing out metabolic waste through the glymphatic system. Poor sleep starves the brain of these processes, maintaining old stress patterns and blocking new learning.

Movement as neurotrophic stimulation

Physical activity increases BDNF (brain-derived neurotrophic factor), insulin sensitivity in the brain, and improves connectivity across neural networks. Sedentary lifestyles are linked not only to metabolic disease, but also to hippocampal shrinkage and impaired emotional regulation.

Breath and nervous system tone

How you breathe daily tells your autonomic nervous system whether it should be in sympathetic (fight-flight) or parasympathetic (rest-repair) dominance. Rapid, shallow breathing is interpreted as a cue for danger, while slow diaphragmatic breathing signals safety.

Social and emotional inputs

Your relationships, social environments, and even the tone of your inner dialogue are neural inputs. Chronic conflict, isolation, or harsh self-talk reinforce limbic patterns of threat and defense. Meaningful connection and laughter literally reshape your amygdala's sensitivity and expand prefrontal regulatory circuits.

The cumulative ffect: Lifestyle as a neural environment

Over days, weeks, and months, these small choices accumulate into a biological climate—one that either:

Reinforces defensive loops (hypervigilance, inflammation, hormonal shutdown), or supports flexibility, resilience, and repair.

In other words, your daily habits are not only sculpting your waistline or cholesterol levels. They are training your nervous system. They are repeatedly telling your brain what to expect from the world—danger or safety, scarcity or abundance, urgency or permission to rest.

Why this matters for regeneration

Neuroplasticity—the brain's ability to reorganize itself by forming new connections—requires both the opportunity and the right conditions. If your mind and body stay locked in micro-states of stress, shallow breathing, late-night scrolling, processed food, and emotional discord, it sends a clear, unified message to your nervous system:

"Stay alert. Stay ready. Now is not the time to rebuild."

But when your lifestyle inputs consistently reinforce signals of safety, nourishment, movement, oxygenation, emotional expression, and calm, your body gets a very different message:

"It is safe to digest. Safe to balance hormones. Safe to repair tissue. Safe to prune old neural pathways and build new ones."

This is how lifestyle functions as a neural modulator, dictating not just whether healing is desired, but whether it is even biologically permitted.

Shaping your inner ecosystem

So much of health is about removing confusion for the nervous system. By aligning your lifestyle inputs—your breath, your food, your relationships, your rest—with the messages of safety and possibility, you create a clear neural environment that promotes:

Improved heart rate variability (HRV)

Better limbic regulation (less chronic fear or anger)

Balanced immune and endocrine outputs

Faster integration of therapeutic changes, whether through hypnosis, frequency work, or conventional medicine

Lifestyle is not just a background factor in healing. It is the soil in which all neurological and biological change takes root.

Nutrition, movement, sleep, and nature as brain signals

How everyday choices directly instruct your nervous system

We tend to see nutrition, exercise, sleep, and time outdoors as lifestyle habits that affect our bodies. But in reality, they function as powerful, continuous streams of information for the brain and nervous system. They are not just background health factors — they are core inputs that regulate how the brain fires, how it rewires, and how the body heals.

In a very real sense, these lifestyle foundations act like instructions that tell your system whether to prioritize growth and regeneration or protection and shutdown.

Nutrition: More than fuel — Molecular messaging for the brain

What we eat doesn't just give us calories; it provides biochemical signals that shape neurotransmitters, brain inflammation levels, and synaptic growth.

Nutrients like omega-3 fatty acids (from fatty fish, flax, walnuts) are essential for building neuronal membranes and reducing microglial overactivation — a key driver of neuroinflammation linked to depression, brain fog, and even neurodegeneration.

Amino acids from proteins are precursors to dopamine, serotonin, GABA, and other neurotransmitters that determine mood, motivation, and calm.

Antioxidants from colorful fruits and vegetables help neutralize free radicals, reducing oxidative stress that can damage neural tissue and accelerate aging.

Conversely, diets high in refined sugar and processed fats contribute to insulin resistance in the brain, promote chronic inflammation, and impair hippocampal function — directly undermining learning and memory.

Every meal is a set of molecular instructions that influences how your brain functions, repairs, and responds to stress.

Movement: A direct stimulus for neuroplasticity

Exercise is not just about muscles or cardiovascular endurance; it's one of the most potent drivers of neuroplastic change we have.

Physical activity increases brain-derived neurotrophic factor (BDNF), often called "fertilizer for the brain," which supports the growth of new neurons and strengthens existing synapses.

It improves insulin sensitivity in the brain, enhancing energy metabolism for cognitive tasks and memory consolidation.

Regular movement also dampens the chronic output of stress hormones, reduces limbic overactivity, and improves functional connectivity between the prefrontal cortex (planning and decision-making) and the amygdala (fear and threat processing).

Even low-intensity activities like walking, gentle yoga, or tai chi send signals of safety and rhythm, training the nervous system to stabilize, downshift hypervigilance, and support cellular repair.

Sleep: Where the brain cleans, sorts, and restores

Sleep is often underappreciated, but it is arguably the most critical period for neurological maintenance and regeneration.

During deep, slow-wave sleep (delta states), the brain's glymphatic system clears out metabolic waste, including beta-amyloid plaques implicated in Alzheimer's disease.

Important neuroplastic processes such as memory consolidation and synaptic pruning happen primarily during REM and non-REM cycles.

Sleep regulates cortisol rhythms and supports balanced immune signaling, reducing systemic inflammation that could otherwise damage both brain and peripheral tissues.

Poor or inconsistent sleep disrupts these cycles, leaving the brain less able to form new connections, less resilient under stress, and more prone to perpetuating maladaptive patterns.

Nature: An ancient signal of safety and regulation

Time spent in natural environments — forests, mountains, the ocean — has profound effects on the brain and autonomic nervous system.

Visual inputs from trees, water, and wide horizons reduce activity in the default mode network (associated with rumination and self-critical thought) and enhance parasympathetic tone.

Phytoncides (compounds released by trees) and the negative ions present in natural spaces lower cortisol, improve mood, and support immune function.

Direct contact with the earth ("grounding" or "earthing") may influence inflammation and redox balance, although the mechanisms are still being investigated.

Even brief exposures — like a 15-minute walk in a park — send the nervous system a clear signal: "You are not under immediate threat. It is safe to rest, digest, and rebuild."

The unifying principle: Lifestyle inputs as neural instructions

All of these lifestyle foundations — nutrition, movement, sleep, and nature — are not simply external routines. They are direct channels of communication with your brain and body, shaping:

How neurons fire and wire together

How the amygdala and limbic system perceive risk

How the hypothalamus sets hormone outputs

How immune cells patrol or inflame tissue

How genes switch on processes for inflammation vs. repair

When these inputs consistently convey safety, nourishment, and rhythm, they lower the brain's perceived need for defense, making space for plasticity, hormonal balance, and cellular regeneration.

Your daily habits are not just keeping your body alive.They are sending moment-by-moment instructions to your nervous system about whether to grow, heal, or hold back.

By consciously shaping these inputs, you turn lifestyle into the most fundamental form of medicine.

How daily habits affect neuroplasticity and healing

Shaping your brain, body, and energy field through everyday choices

Healing is not simply the result of a powerful one-time intervention. It is the outcome of repeated signals that guide your nervous system to either maintain old defensive patterns or open to regeneration. This means that your daily habits — seemingly small choices — have profound power to sculpt your brain, recalibrate your body, and even influence the subtle energy fields that surround and interpenetrate your tissues.

Neuroplasticity is the brain's capacity to rewire itself by forming new neural connections and pruning away outdated ones. This plasticity is not a given; it is exquisitely sensitive to the environment you create through your thoughts, behaviors, sensory experiences, and physiological rhythms.

Likewise, the body's capacity to repair — from micro-level cellular turnover to large-scale immune recalibration — is continuously modulated by these same inputs.

The daily dance: Habits as ongoing neural instructions

Every habit is a repetitive piece of information that instructs your nervous system on how to calibrate itself.

When you wake up and immediately check stressful news or social feeds, your amygdala is primed for vigilance.

When you sit under artificial light all day, your suprachiasmatic nucleus (brain clock) receives confused signals about circadian rhythms, disrupting sleep hormones and repair processes.

When you stay indoors, away from green light spectrums and natural electromagnetic inputs, your entire neuroendocrine-immune axis misses out on grounding, regulating cues.

When you breathe shallowly at your desk, your vagus nerve receives a subtle message to prepare for fight-or-flight.

Conversely, simple choices like:

Going outside in natural morning light,

Taking slow, deep breaths that extend your exhale,

Moving your body rhythmically,

Nourishing yourself with omega-3s, polyphenols, and high-antioxidant foods,

And immersing yourself in healing sounds and frequencies...

...all send powerful signals of safety, rhythm, and replenishment. They literally tell your nervous system, "You can step out of defense. Now is a good time to repair."

Neuroplasticity Needs More Than Novelty — It Needs the Right Environment

The brain changes all the time, but the quality of change depends on the context you create.

Chronic stress — whether from lifestyle mismatch, emotional strain, or internalized hypervigilance — increases excitatory neurotransmitters like glutamate and stress hormones like cortisol. This environment encourages the brain to reinforce old survival-based wiring, strengthening circuits related to threat detection and bodily shutdown.

In contrast, when you build a lifestyle filled with calm, restorative, joyful experiences, you increase neurotrophic factors (like BDNF), improve synaptic pruning, and enhance integration between the prefrontal cortex (rational thought) and limbic system (emotion). This allows for healthy rewiring — making new patterns of thought, feeling, and immune response possible.

Sound baths and vibration bowls: Energizing body and field

Among the most fascinating tools to support both neuroplastic healing and your subtle energy field are sound baths and vibration bowls.

How They Work

Sound baths typically use instruments like crystal bowls, Himalayan singing bowls, gongs, and chimes that create rich layers of vibration and frequency. These sounds do more than please the ear:

They produce oscillating waves that penetrate through the skin, fascia, and even cellular structures, subtly entraining them.

Research shows sound can help shift brainwave patterns from high-alert beta into slower alpha, theta, and even delta states, the same states associated with deep healing, memory reconsolidation, and tissue repair.

Impact on the body's energy field

Beyond measurable neurology, many traditions and emerging studies explore how vibration from bowls and gongs harmonizes the body's electromagnetic field (often referred to as the biofield). This subtle field is thought to play a role in guiding cellular communication and maintaining system-wide coherence.

Practitioners and clients alike report experiences such as:

A sense of internal alignment or tingling "clearing" sensations

Emotional releases as old patterns loosen

Enhanced clarity or a gentle euphoria following sessions

Clinical and Wellness Benefits

Regular use of sound baths or vibration bowls has been associated with:

Reduced perceived stress and anxiety

Improved heart rate variability (a marker of autonomic flexibility)

Better sleep quality and digestion (via vagal regulation)

Relief of tension patterns in muscles and fascia

Integrating This Into Daily Neuroplastic Healing

Just like diet or movement, intentional use of sound is a lifestyle input — a daily choice that signals your nervous system to synchronize, downshift defense modes, and open to renewal.

Examples of integrating these tools:

Ending your day with a 15-minute sound bath to transition from high beta to restorative theta before sleep.

Using a small vibration bowl to start your meditation, aligning breath and brain rhythms.

Pairing gentle bowl sessions with breathwork to deepen parasympathetic activation.

Even short moments of humming or chanting can create resonance in the vagus nerve and chest cavity, reinforcing calm.

The cumulative message

Your daily habits — what you eat, how you move, when you sleep, how you breathe, what sounds and environments you bathe in — are not trivial. They are the software continuously programming your brain and the bioelectrical signals orchestrating your body.

They train your nervous system to decide each day whether to remain cautious, inflamed, and braced for threat — or to explore, repair, and regenerate.

Healing is not only about the interventions we seek; it is about the micro-signals we send to our brain and body all day long.

Every choice is a new instruction:

"Keep surviving" or "Start thriving."

Creating an internal healing ecosystem

Synchronizing lifestyle with trance therapy for lasting regeneration

One of the most overlooked truths in modern health is that healing is rarely achieved by a single technique, treatment, or insight. It emerges from an internal ecosystem—a living network of thoughts, emotions, biochemical states, electrical rhythms, and subtle energetic patterns that either nurture regeneration or keep the body locked in defense.

If trance therapy (such as clinical hypnosis) is the focused portal into subconscious reprogramming, your daily lifestyle is the ongoing climate that determines whether those new patterns truly take root.

In this sense, lifestyle is not secondary; it is the environment in which all deeper therapeutic work either flourishes or struggles to survive.

Why synchronization matters?

Imagine guiding the subconscious into powerful states of receptivity and installing healing instructions through deep trance—only to spend the rest of the day:

Consuming inflammatory foods,

Staying sedentary under artificial light,

Reactivating vigilance through constant digital input,

Breathing shallowly,

or simmering in unprocessed stress.

Each of these habits quietly reinforces the very neural circuits and hormonal outputs that hypnosis or meditation seeks to recalibrate.

In contrast, when lifestyle and trance work are synchronized, they send a unified message to your brain and body:

"It is safe now. Repair is permitted. Balance is supported."

This synergy doesn't just accelerate change—it stabilizes it, turning temporary improvements into lasting transformation.

The internal healing ecosystem: What it involves

Creating an ecosystem inside your body and mind that naturally supports regeneration involves orchestrating several layers of input:

Nutrition

Choosing foods rich in omega-3s, polyphenols, antioxidants, minerals, and diverse plant fibers reduces neuroinflammation, supports gut-brain signaling, and provides the raw materials for neurotransmitter balance. This biochemical calm sets the stage for deeper nervous system recalibration.

Movement

Rhythmic, joyful movement—walking, gentle stretching, dance, mindful exercise—improves lymphatic flow, enhances neurotrophic factors like BDNF, and signals to the limbic system that it is safe to shift out of defense.

Sleep and circadian integrity

Deep, consistent sleep allows the brain to consolidate new neural patterns laid down in trance work, detoxify waste, balance cortisol rhythms, and reinforce the new "healing software" you are installing.

Nature and grounding

Time spent in natural environments harmonizes the body's electromagnetic fields, soothes amygdala reactivity, and re-establishes the body's relationship to natural circadian and magnetic cycles. Even short daily exposures can profoundly support autonomic and emotional regulation.

Breath and internal rhythm

Slow, diaphragmatic breathing practiced throughout the day builds on trance work by keeping the vagus nerve engaged, maintaining parasympathetic tone, and preventing the mind from slipping back into shallow, rapid stress patterns.

Integrating healing frequencies and vibrational therapy

An especially powerful adjunct to this ecosystem is the deliberate use of sound and vibrational inputs—tools that work below cognitive awareness, directly influencing the body's electrical and energetic systems.

This includes:

Sound baths with vibration bowls (such as crystal or Himalayan singing bowls), which emit frequencies that entrain both brainwaves and the body's subtle energy field. Many report sensations of "internal clearing," reduced tension, and emotional release—effects backed by emerging studies on heart rate variability, limbic calming, and reduced cortisol.

Specialized healing frequency tracks, like those offered in collaboration between LifeBoss Health and the HypnoCell® methodology, designed to be paired with trance sessions. These frequencies help maintain theta and delta rhythms even outside formal hypnosis, reinforcing neural recalibration and helping the body "stay tuned" to a state of repair.

Personal vocal toning or humming, which stimulates the vagus nerve and creates resonant waves in the chest cavity, bridging conscious practice and subconscious soothing.

Bringing it all together: A truly regenerative terrain

When trance therapy is layered into a lifestyle that supports the same neurological and biological goals, healing moves from episodic to systemic.

Hypnosis and deep guided states directly reprogram maladaptive subconscious patterns, making room for new instructions.

Nutrition, sleep, breath, movement, nature, and vibration maintain a biochemical, electrical, and emotional climate where those instructions are continually reinforced.

This holistic approach does not leave your transformation vulnerable to relapse from daily contradictions. Instead, it builds an internal ecosystem where every part of life supports the nervous system in choosing growth, repair, and balance over vigilance and shutdown.

Healing is never only what happens in the session.It is the ongoing dialogue between your deepest mind and the environment you create for it every day.

By aligning lifestyle with inner therapeutic work, you turn regeneration from possibility into probability.

Chapter 8

The practice of self-hypnosis and regenerative meditation

One of the most empowering aspects of healing is realizing that it is not limited to what happens in a therapy office or medical clinic. True regeneration often depends on what you can cultivate within yourself, day after day, in the spaces between formal treatments.

Self-hypnosis and regenerative meditation are two of the most effective tools to guide your brain and nervous system into states that support profound change. They allow you to consciously access the same deep neuroplastic and autonomic environments that clinical hypnosis or guided frequency work targets—giving you the power to continue reprogramming your patterns, even when you are alone.

These practices are not mystical or complex. They are evidence-based techniques for entering targeted states of brain activity (alpha, theta, and delta), reducing limbic overactivity, calming the stress axis, and embedding new neural pathways that favor healing.

Why These Practices Are So Potent for Regeneration

The body and brain do not heal effectively in states of defense. Chronic sympathetic dominance—high alert, shallow breathing, muscle tension, fragmented attention—prioritizes survival, not repair.

Self-hypnosis and regenerative meditation do the opposite. They:

Shift brainwaves from high beta (anxious, scattered thinking) into slower alpha and theta, which open subconscious doors and promote calm integration.

Lower cortisol and regulate the hypothalamic-pituitary-adrenal (HPA) axis, reducing systemic inflammation.

Activate parasympathetic dominance, increasing vagal tone, improving digestion, fertility, immune clarity, and cellular repair.

Provide the repetition necessary for neuroplasticity—gradually overwriting old circuits tied to hypervigilance, chronic pain, or emotional shutdown.

With consistent practice, these techniques teach your nervous system a new baseline—one oriented toward safety, coherence, and restoration.

What's the Difference Between the Two?

Self-Hypnosis

Self-hypnosis is a structured process where you guide yourself into a focused, trance-like state—often using breath, body relaxation, and intentional suggestion. It typically involves:

Identifying a core area of change (e.g., "I want to retrain my response to pain," or "I want my body to remember it's safe to heal.")

Using scripts, imagery, or carefully chosen affirmations delivered in a rhythmic, absorbing way.

Embedding the new narrative or sensory reality deeply into subconscious pathways.

Because it's suggestive and directive, self-hypnosis is particularly powerful for targeted reprogramming—like breaking a chronic symptom loop or installing new instructions for the immune system.

Regenerative Meditation

Regenerative meditation is typically less directive, creating a spacious inner field where the nervous system can naturally recalibrate. Practices might include:

Body scanning with loving awareness.

Visualizing light or vibrational energy moving through organs or tissues.

Sitting in spacious, breath-focused stillness that allows protective patterns to dissolve on their own.

Letting imagery or spontaneous "healing stories" emerge from within.

This approach emphasizes being rather than doing, inviting deeper levels of unconscious processing, emotional integration, and subtle energetic shifts.

The Synergy of Both Practices

Used together, self-hypnosis and regenerative meditation offer both precision and spaciousness—the intentional reprogramming of maladaptive loops, plus the open nurturing space in which new circuits stabilize and deepen.

For example:

You might start with a short self-hypnosis session focused on reframing a specific pattern (like calming digestive reactivity or releasing an old trauma imprint), then finish with 10 minutes of silent, breath-led meditation, allowing your body to integrate the new state without pushing.

Long-Term Neuroplastic Effects

Over time, these practices:

Strengthen synaptic pathways associated with calm, safety, and pleasure.

Weaken old circuits tied to hypervigilance, rumination, or somatic distress.

Improve the coherence of brain regions like the prefrontal cortex (executive function) and amygdala (emotional memory), leading to more balanced responses.

Help establish heart-brain synchronization, supporting emotional regulation and reducing chronic stress chemistry.

Your system literally learns a new normal—one in which healing is no longer an exception but a baseline biological priority.

Supporting tools: Frequency and vibration

Many people find these inner practices even more powerful when paired with gentle frequency-based supports—such as sound baths, vibration bowls, or specialized healing frequencies (including programs offered through LifeBoss Health in collaboration with HypnoCell®, designed to entrain brainwave states and reinforce cellular resonance). These external cues guide the nervous system into deep theta and delta more quickly, amplifying the effects of your inner work.

Healing is not something that only happens to you.It's something your mind and body learn to do—through repetition, safety, and new instructions.

Self-hypnosis and regenerative meditation give you the ability to become an active participant in your own reprogramming.

Protocols to safely induce self-hypnosis

Guiding yourself into the brain states where healing and rewiring occur

Self-hypnosis is not about "giving up control" or forcing the mind into a blank state. It is a structured, intentional way to guide yourself into an altered state of consciousness where your brain shifts from high-alert problem solving into slower, integrative brainwave patterns (alpha, theta, and even delta).

In these states, the critical, analytical mind softens, allowing direct communication with subconscious and unconscious processes—where the deepest drivers of pain, inflammation, immune imbalance, or emotional reactivity reside.

When practiced with care, self-hypnosis is one of the safest, most accessible ways to facilitate neuroplastic reprogramming, emotional release, and somatic recalibration.

Why a Protocol Matters?

Because self-hypnosis works by bypassing your usual mental filters, it is important to have a gentle, clear structure. This:

Keeps the nervous system feeling safe and supported (not startled or overwhelmed).

Ensures suggestions are framed positively and ethically, aligned with your genuine healing goals.

Helps maintain enough conscious awareness to observe shifts without resistance or fear.

A reliable protocol becomes like a mental runway—guiding you smoothly into trance, supporting you while there, and helping you return grounded and calm.

A simple, repeatable self-hypnosis protocol

This is a foundational structure you can adapt to virtually any goal—whether easing chronic tension, calming gut or immune reactivity, or gently rewriting an old emotional pattern.

1. Prepare the space and intention

Find a quiet place where you won't be disturbed for 15–30 minutes.

Sit or lie comfortably, keeping your spine supported if seated.

Set a clear, gentle intention, e.g.:

"I am guiding myself to a calm, receptive state where my mind and body can safely explore healing."

Silence notifications and, if you like, play soft background sound such as nature tracks or low-frequency tones.

2. Progressive physical relaxation

Begin by closing your eyes and taking three slow, deep breaths.

Let your attention move through your body, from head to toes, lightly inviting each area to release.

Example inner language:

"My forehead is soft... my jaw releases... my shoulders drop... my belly loosens..."

This process helps signal the parasympathetic nervous system to take the lead, lowering heart rate, blood pressure, and muscle guarding.

3. Entering focused absorption (induction

Choose a simple focus point to deepen the trance. Options include:

Counting down slowly from 10 to 1, imagining yourself sinking deeper with each number.

Visualizing descending a gentle staircase or floating deeper into warm water.

Repeating a soft phrase like:

"Deeper, calmer, safer..."

If your mind wanders, simply notice and return to your chosen anchor. You are not trying to force blankness—just inviting single-pointed focus.

4. Delivering healing suggestions or imagery

Once you feel more spacious (time may seem slower, body heavier or lighter, thoughts quieter), introduce your core healing idea.

This could be:

A visual scene of your immune system gently balancing, tissues knitting together, or energy flowing freely.

A verbal suggestion, repeated softly:

"It is safe for my body to restore. Every cell knows how to regenerate."

A symbolic metaphor, such as a light clearing dark clouds or roots growing deep and stable.

Keep your language positive, present-tense, and gentle. Your subconscious works best with imagery and feeling, not rigid commands.

5. Integration and Gentle Return

When ready (often after 10–20 minutes), slowly count up from 1 to 5 or imagine yourself rising back up the same staircase.Gently stretch or wiggle your fingers and toes. Take a deep breath, open your eyes, and sit for a moment before moving.

Reinforce the session by acknowledging:

"I have given my mind and body new instructions today. They are now beginning to take root."

Safety Considerations

Always keep self-hypnosis framed as an exploration, not force. If you become emotionally overwhelmed, gently shift to simply observing your breath until calm returns.

Avoid using negative phrases like "I won't feel pain." Instead use, "I am inviting calm and ease."

If dealing with significant trauma memories, work alongside a skilled clinical hypnotist or trauma therapist who can safely hold space.

Supporting Tools: Breath, Sound, and Frequency

To deepen and stabilize the trance:

Try slow 4-7-8 breathing (inhale 4, hold 7, exhale 8).

Use soft binaural beats or vibration bowls to entrain your brain into theta.

Some specialized healing frequency tracks (such as those offered through LifeBoss Health collaborations) can maintain a resonance that supports deeper relaxation and subtle cellular coherence.

The Power of Repetition

Neuroplastic change relies on repeated, emotionally charged experience. Practicing self-hypnosis a few times a week—even for just 15 minutes—gradually builds new neural defaults, teaching your system to return to states of calm regulation and regenerative readiness.

Self-hypnosis is not about forcing healing. It's about creating the internal conditions where your mind and body remember how.

With each gentle session, you lay down the pathways for ease, balance, and true renewal.

Daily scripts and anchor techniques

Simple tools to reinforce neuroplastic change and create consistent healing signals

While deep trance sessions and guided hypnosis play a critical role in accessing subconscious patterns, true transformation is most powerfully cemented through daily, repeated reinforcement.

This is where short scripts (mini self-hypnosis or focused suggestion sessions) and anchor techniques (sensory or physical cues tied to a desired state) become invaluable. They work together to keep your brain and body consistently receiving the same message of safety, possibility, and repair — day after day, until it becomes a new default.

Why short, frequent inputs matter

Neuroplasticity doesn't rely only on intensity — it thrives on frequency and consistency.

Just as a muscle strengthens through repeated lifts rather than a single heavy strain, neural circuits become more efficient and automatic through small, daily rehearsals.

This regular repetition stabilizes the "healing software" introduced in longer sessions, preventing the brain from easily slipping back into old protective loops.

Daily scripts: Quick neural rehearsals for healing

Think of a daily script as a short, focused self-hypnosis or intentional meditation, typically 2–5 minutes long. It uses your voice and imagination to guide the brain into a lightly receptive state and then embeds targeted suggestions.

What a script looks like

A daily script includes:

Brief centering:

One or two deep breaths, relaxing your shoulders and face.

Simple drop-in cue:

"As I close my eyes, I let my mind settle, just for a moment."

Targeted suggestion or imagery:

"My body knows how to heal. Every cell remembers balance. My breath is guiding this process now."

Gentle closing:

"These new instructions are settling in, continuing on their own. I can return to them anytime."

Examples of daily scripts

For immune & cellular repair:

"With each gentle breath, my body shifts into regeneration. My immune system is clear, wise, balanced. Repair happens easily, naturally, without force."

For calming pain loops:

"As my breath flows deeper, I invite softness into every area of tension. My brain is learning new patterns of ease. It is safe to release."

For emotional safety & regulation:

"Right now, I am safe. My heart beats steadily. My mind can rest. My body can recalibrate, here and now."

Anchor techniques: Wiring healing to the senses

Anchoring is a classical hypnotic and neuro-linguistic tool that links a physical sensation or sensory cue to a desired internal state. Over time, simply triggering the anchor can bring back that state automatically, bypassing lengthy mental processing.

How to set an anchor

Enter a lightly relaxed state — after a few breaths or your short daily script.

Focus on a felt sense of calm, strength, or whatever quality you're installing.

Pair it with a deliberate sensory gesture, like:

Gently pressing thumb and forefinger together

Placing your hand on your heart

Exhaling with a soft audible "humm" sound

Repeat this pairing several times. Your brain starts wiring the physical cue to the internal state.

Benefits of anchors

Allows you to re-trigger calm or confidence on demand, even in stressful settings.

Creates a tangible, sensory pathway for subconscious states—bridging mind and body.

Reinforces the new neural circuits, making them more dominant over time.

How to Integrate daily scripts & anchors

Use your short script in the morning to prime your nervous system, and again in the evening to help consolidate the new pathways during sleep.

Reinforce throughout the day by firing your anchor—like pressing your fingertips lightly together when you start to feel stressed or distracted.

Keep scripts gentle, present tense, and emotionally resonant. Avoid forcing. The subconscious responds to invitation and imagery, not pressure.

Healing is not only created in big breakthrough moments.It is built in tiny, repeated signals that teach your brain, body, and heart a new way to be.

Bonus tip: Stack with breath or sound

Try pairing your anchor with a slow exhale or a soft "mmm" vibration in the chest.

This enhances vagal activation, stabilizes the autonomic shift, and embeds the neural association even deeper.

Using visualization and somatic cues to amplify brain–body connection

Activating the mind's power to influence physiology, rewire patterns, and enhance healing

One of the most remarkable insights from neuroscience and psychophysiology is that the brain does not perfectly distinguish between what is vividly imagined and what is actually happening. This means that targeted visualization—combined with somatic cues (physical sensations and movements)—can dramatically influence how your body responds, right down to immune, endocrine, and cellular processes.

By consciously engaging imagery and bodily awareness, you can strengthen the communication loop between mind and body, guiding your nervous system toward states that favor restoration, resilience, and neuroplastic change.

Daily scripts and anchor techniques

Simple tools to reinforce neuroplastic change and create consistent healing signals

While deep trance sessions and guided hypnosis play a critical role in accessing subconscious patterns, true transformation is most powerfully cemented through daily, repeated reinforcement.

This is where short scripts (mini self-hypnosis or focused suggestion sessions) and anchor techniques (sensory or physical cues tied to a desired state) become invaluable. They work together to keep your brain and body consistently receiving the same message of safety, possibility, and repair — day after day, until it becomes a new default.

Why short, frequent inputs matter

Neuroplasticity doesn't rely only on intensity — it thrives on frequency and consistency.

Just as a muscle strengthens through repeated lifts rather than a single heavy strain, neural circuits become more efficient and automatic through small, daily rehearsals.

This regular repetition stabilizes the "healing software" introduced in longer sessions, preventing the brain from easily slipping back into old protective loops.

Daily scripts: Quick neural rehearsals for healing

Think of a daily script as a short, focused self-hypnosis or intentional meditation, typically 2–5 minutes long. It uses your voice and imagination to guide the brain into a lightly receptive state and then embeds targeted suggestions.

What a script looks like

A daily script includes:

Brief centering:

One or two deep breaths, relaxing your shoulders and face.

Simple drop-in cue:

"As I close my eyes, I let my mind settle, just for a moment."

Targeted suggestion or imagery:

"My body knows how to heal. Every cell remembers balance. My breath is guiding this process now."

Gentle closing:

"These new instructions are settling in, continuing on their own. I can return to them anytime."

Examples of daily scripts

For immune & cellular repair:

"With each gentle breath, my body shifts into regeneration. My immune system is clear, wise, balanced. Repair happens easily, naturally, without force."

For calming pain loops:

"As my breath flows deeper, I invite softness into every area of tension. My brain is learning new patterns of ease. It is safe to release."

For emotional safety & regulation:

"Right now, I am safe. My heart beats steadily. My mind can rest. My body can recalibrate, here and now."

Anchor Techniques: Wiring Healing to the Senses

Anchoring is a classical hypnotic and neuro-linguistic tool that links a physical sensation or sensory cue to a desired internal state. Over time, simply triggering the anchor can bring back that state automatically, bypassing lengthy mental processing.

How to set an anchor

Enter a lightly relaxed state — after a few breaths or your short daily script.

Focus on a felt sense of calm, strength, or whatever quality you're installing.

Pair it with a deliberate sensory gesture, like:

Gently pressing thumb and forefinger together

Placing your hand on your heart

Exhaling with a soft audible "humm" sound

Repeat this pairing several times. Your brain starts wiring the physical cue to the internal state.

Benefits of anchors

Allows you to re-trigger calm or confidence on demand, even in stressful settings.

Creates a tangible, sensory pathway for subconscious states—bridging mind and body.

Reinforces the new neural circuits, making them more dominant over time.

How to integrate daily scripts & anchors

Use your short script in the morning to prime your nervous system, and again in the evening to help consolidate the new pathways during sleep.

Reinforce throughout the day by firing your anchor—like pressing your fingertips lightly together when you start to feel stressed or distracted.

Keep scripts gentle, present tense, and emotionally resonant. Avoid forcing. The subconscious responds to invitation and imagery, not pressure.

Healing is not only created in big breakthrough moments.It is built in tiny, repeated signals that teach your brain, body, and heart a new way to be.

Bonus tip: Stack with breath or sound

Try pairing your anchor with a slow exhale or a soft "mmm" vibration in the chest.

This enhances vagal activation, stabilizes the autonomic shift, and embeds the neural association even deeper.

Using visualization and somatic cues to amplify brain–body connection

Activating the mind's power to influence physiology, rewire patterns, and enhance healing

One of the most remarkable insights from neuroscience and psychophysiology is that the brain does not perfectly distinguish between what is vividly imagined and what is actually happening. This means that targeted visualization—combined with somatic cues (physical sensations and movements)—can dramatically influence how your body responds, right down to immune, endocrine, and cellular processes.

By consciously engaging imagery and bodily awareness, you can strengthen the communication loop between mind and body, guiding your nervous system toward states that favor restoration, resilience, and neuroplastic change.

Why visualization works

Studies using fMRI and PET scans have shown that when people imagine moving a limb, experiencing a sensation, or seeing a calming scene, the same neural circuits activate as when they physically do it.

Mental imagery of walking lights up motor planning areas.

Imagining a comforting touch can reduce amygdala reactivity and lower cortisol.

Visualizing inflammation cooling or tissues knitting together engages sensory cortex regions, which then feed back to autonomic outputs.

This means visualization can train the brain to expect and support healing, gently reprogramming it to prioritize growth and repair instead of chronic defense.

Why somatic cues enhance the effect

Adding somatic (body-based) cues—like breath awareness, muscle release, gentle touch, or even posture changes—amplifies the brain's sense that the imagery is **real**.

When you pair an image of calm expansion with a slow exhale, the vagus nerve is stimulated, reinforcing parasympathetic states.

Placing a hand on your heart while visualizing warmth or light there sends tactile signals that support the mental picture.

Even subtle shifts—like softening the jaw or dropping the shoulders—send feedback to the brainstem that confirms "We are safe now," encouraging deeper autonomic shifts.

Practical Example

To ease chronic tension or pain:

Close your eyes and take several slow breaths, imagining each inhale carrying in light or a gentle soothing mist.

With each exhale, visualize the area of discomfort softening, the edges blurring, or cooling like ice melting into calm water.

Place a hand over the area or on your chest, lightly stroking or pressing in rhythm with the breath.

Repeat an internal phrase such as:

"My body knows how to ease and mend. I'm guiding it there now."

This layered approach of imagery + somatic input enhances neuroplastic learning, teaching the nervous system to respond differently over time.

The role of self-practice vs. guided work

While self-visualization and body-focused meditation are powerful daily tools, it's also important to understand that they have natural limits.

On your own, you can access light to moderate trance states, sufficient to influence daily stress patterns, gently lower pain or calm the gut, and reinforce new beliefs.

However, many of the deepest subconscious imprints and defensive neural loops resist change precisely because they were formed under intense emotional conditions (trauma, fear, chronic overwhelm).

A skilled practitioner—especially in guided hypnosis or therapeutic visualization—can:

Navigate past conscious barriers more quickly.

Tailor imagery and somatic prompts in real time to the subtle signals your body and subconscious reveal.

Work with metaphor and layered suggestion to bypass surface resistance, achieving levels of neural engagement that often take much longer to reach alone.

This doesn't mean guided work is "better," but it can often accelerate change, unlock hidden emotional or somatic patterns, and help safely integrate complex memories or protective responses that self-practice might struggle to fully address.

Why this matters for healing and regeneration

At its core, visualization paired with somatic cues is about building a dialogue between the mind and the physical body.

It replaces vague "hope to heal" with specific, rehearsed sensory experiences of what healing might feel like—preparing your brain and body to embody that state.

It shifts top-down processing (conscious expectation) and bottom-up processing (bodily signals) into alignment, creating coherence that favors calm, balanced, repair-focused physiology.

Over time, these practices literally reshape how your brain predicts your body's state, weakening old threat circuits and strengthening new pathways tied to safety, ease, and vitality.

Visualization and somatic cueing are not just mental exercises.They are rehearsals for your biology, teaching your brain and body how to move beyond survival—and remember what it means to truly heal.

Rebuilding resilience, focus, and calm

Training your brain and body to recover strength, adaptability, and inner peace

Healing isn't just about resolving symptoms or overcoming a crisis. It's about restoring the deeper qualities that allow you to meet life's challenges without being overwhelmed—the qualities of resilience, sustained attention, and calm inner regulation.

These are not just abstract personality traits. They are neurobiological capacities, housed in the way your brain circuits fire, how your nervous system toggles between vigilance and rest, and how your endocrine and immune systems interpret your internal world.

Even if you've felt worn down by chronic stress, illness, emotional shock, or prolonged uncertainty, these capacities are not permanently lost. They can be rebuilt through intentional practices that retrain your brain and body to respond from a place of steadiness instead of chronic defense.

Resilience: More than mental toughness

True resilience is not about pushing through at any cost. It is about flexibility—your nervous system's ability to adaptively move between states of alertness and recovery.

When you're resilient:

Your brain can assess situations with perspective, not just reflex.

Your heart rate variability (HRV) reflects a healthy interplay between sympathetic (action) and parasympathetic (repair) systems.

Your immune system stays balanced, neither suppressed under chronic stress nor hyper-reactive.

Your emotional responses can rise when needed, then settle back to baseline without lingering fear or hypervigilance.

Many people mistakenly believe they lack resilience because they feel easily rattled or exhausted. Often, these are the signs of a system that has simply been stuck too long in survival mode—something highly trainable with consistent, targeted inputs.

Rebuilding Focus: Restoring Directed Attention and Cognitive Clarity

Chronic stress, trauma, inflammation, and even persistent emotional burdens can disrupt prefrontal cortex function, the brain's center for focus, planning, and measured decision-making. This is why people often report:

"My mind jumps around constantly."

"I can't finish what I start."

"I lose track of what I was doing halfway through."

Rebuilding focus is not about straining harder. It's about:

Calming limbic (emotional) hyperactivity so the prefrontal cortex can do its job.

Using breath and gentle movement to balance neurotransmitters like dopamine and acetylcholine, which govern attention and motivation.

Practicing short intervals of intentional mental engagement—meditation, visualization, or mindful tasks—to strengthen attentional circuits like you would a muscle.

Cultivating Calm: Repatterning the Default Set Point

Calm is not the absence of challenges. It is the nervous system's ability to return to baseline after activation.

In a healthy pattern, you feel a wave of alertness in response to a problem, then the system resets once the moment passes.

In a dysregulated state, the wave never fully recedes, keeping cortisol, inflammatory markers, and hypervigilance elevated.

Calm becomes a trained default through practices that repetitively signal safety:

Slow, diaphragmatic breathing that lengthens the exhale, directly activating the vagus nerve.

Gentle visualization paired with physical cues (like hand on heart or soothing touch) that teach the brain to associate calm with sensory experience.

Exposure to environments that reduce limbic firing—nature, certain sounds, even soft lighting.

The neuroplastic path: How you rebuild all three together

What's striking is that resilience, focus, and calm are interlinked outcomes of the same neuroplastic rewiring process.

When you practice calming breath and visualization, you lower limbic dominance. This frees up prefrontal resources for focus.

As your attention stabilizes, you feel more capable, which enhances resilience—less mental energy wasted on scattered fear.

As resilience grows, everyday stresses become easier to absorb and bounce back from, reinforcing calm.

The more consistently you engage in practices that cultivate these states, the more your brain shifts from patterns of chronic defense to patterns of adaptive, restorative processing. Over time, this isn't just what you do—it's how your system begins to automatically respond.

Simple daily signals to train resilience, focus, and calm

Breath: Try 5 minutes of extending your exhale to twice the length of your inhale. This downshifts your autonomic tone, teaching your system calm.

Mini-focus intervals: Spend short bursts (even 2–3 minutes) reading something absorbing, doing a puzzle, or practicing slow drawing. This anchors attentional circuits.

Body reassurance: Lightly stroke your chest or abdomen while repeating a soft phrase like "I'm safe right now. It's okay to let go."

Nature micro-dose: Even 5–10 minutes outside, feeling sun on skin or looking at trees, reduces amygdala activation and resets your internal clock.

Healing is not only about removing pain or stress. It's about building the inner strength to meet life with steadiness, clarity, and a nervous system that knows how to come home to calm.

· · · ● · ● · · ·

Chapter 9

The resilient brain – Real stories of regeneration

Healing is often described in terms of lab values, protocols, or theoretical models. But the most powerful testament to the brain's capacity for regeneration comes through the lived experiences of people who have walked through pain, uncertainty, or chronic dysfunction—and emerged transformed.

These are not stories of "perfect cures," nor of bypassing the complexities of medical care. They are stories of ordinary nervous systems doing something extraordinary: recalibrating under the right conditions to reclaim balance, reduce suffering, and rewire patterns that once seemed fixed.

They reveal what neuroscience continues to affirm:

The brain is not static.

The body is not broken.

Given the right internal state and repeated signals of safety and possibility, profound repair and functional improvement are not only possible—they are biologically expected.

Patient stories and cases using the HypnoCell® method

Each of these brief portraits is based on composites of clinical observations, reflecting realistic patterns of progress. They demonstrate the varied and often surprising ways the mind and nervous system respond when engaged through safe, precise, and repeated neuroplastic work.

Case 1: From Chronic Digestive Turmoil to Calm Gut-Brain Harmony

Patient: Carolina, 38, marketing consultant, years of IBS with bloating, cramping, unpredictable flares.

History: Tried multiple elimination diets, probiotics, and medications with partial relief. Stress always made it worse. She'd begun avoiding travel or social events, fearing embarrassing symptoms.

Approach:

Introduced a foundational gut-calming lifestyle routine: slow eating, warm cooked meals, walks after lunch.

Combined with sound-based vagal toning sessions and daily self-hypnosis focused on "rewriting" the gut's hyper-reactivity.

In guided HypnoCell® sessions, uncovered deep subconscious associations of the gut as a "holding zone for worry," dating back to childhood. Used somatic imagery to reassign the gut's role from stress storage to gentle digestion.

Outcome:

Within 6 weeks, fewer urgent episodes, increased confidence to leave the house.

Reported feeling "neutral" about digestion for the first time in years—a profound shift from daily dread.

Not symptom-free every day, but her baseline resilience dramatically improved, with flare-ups lasting hours instead of days.

Case 2: Easing neuroinflammation and migraines through repatterning

Patient: Matteo, 44, engineer, lifelong high performer with increasing migraines, light sensitivity, and "brain fog" that conventional neurologic workup could not fully resolve.

History: MRI clear, lifestyle healthy by most measures, but episodes worsening. Felt ashamed to admit fear of decline.

Approach:

Focused on establishing robust sleep and morning light exposure to stabilize circadian signals.

Paired evening regenerative meditations with low-frequency sound to encourage delta dominance before bed.

In HypnoCell® sessions, uncovered subconscious "permission" issues—his brain had learned hypervigilance as a means to succeed, equating relaxation with loss of edge.

Used deep trance imagery to retrain his brain to see calm focus as an upgrade, not a liability.

Outcome:

By 3 months, migraine frequency cut by more than half, cognitive clarity improved, needed less caffeine.

Most meaningfully, he described "liking his own mind again" and trusting that if a migraine started, it didn't mean catastrophic collapse.

Case 3: Rebalancing autoimmune reactivity

Patient: Lara, 52, teacher, diagnosed with an autoimmune thyroid condition (Hashimoto's) ten years earlier, on stable medication but still plagued by exhaustion, skin flare-ups, and deep internal agitation.

History: Labs often stable, yet she felt something "locked inside still battling." Emotional triggers or even minor stress would bring symptom flares.

Approach:

Integrated gentle breath-led somatic practices to cue parasympathetic regulation daily.

Used specialized healing frequencies (a collaboration with LifeBoss Health and HypnoCell®) to help reinforce theta states during self-guided trance.

In deeper subconscious work, traced lingering autoimmune hyperalertness to a lifetime of feeling over-responsible. Through hypnotic re-scripting, her nervous system practiced the concept: "I can be supported. I do not have to remain on guard."

Outcome:

Reported more consistent energy, less skin reactivity under stress, and an unexpected side effect: lighter, more spontaneous emotions.

Stated, "My body doesn't feel like it's at war with me all the time anymore."

Case 4: Emotional trauma and chronic Muscular Guarding

Patient: Nabil, 31, tech consultant, chronic neck and shoulder tightness that no amount of massage, stretching, or posture correction could resolve.

History: Low-level anxiety most of his life. Survived a car accident in adolescence, "walked away fine," but ever since felt hyper-alert, with shallow breathing and frequent startling.

Approach:

Began with simple breath and micro-movement practices to reduce baseline tension.

Progressed into targeted HypnoCell® trance sessions uncovering somatic memories from the accident. Used visualization to "complete" the defensive motion frozen in his body.

Installed daily anchor techniques—gently pressing his sternum and breathing while repeating, "It's okay to soften now."

Outcome:

Within 8 weeks, noticed waking up without jaw clenching, shoulders no longer painfully high by afternoon.

Said he felt "like the volume dial on life turned down a bit — but in a good way."

Became more emotionally available, describing it as "getting my bandwidth back."

The bigger picture

None of these people experienced a fairy-tale flip from illness to perfect health. Their stories are about incremental shifts in how their brains interpreted signals, how their bodies chose to respond, and how their inner environments gradually prioritized healing over protection.

Their cases stand as living proof that resilience is not something mystical — it is the natural outcome when mind and body receive consistent, reinforcing instructions to move from vigilance to repair.

The brain is resilient by design.

With the right inner conditions, it learns to reorganize. The stories of real people remind us: repair is written into your biology—your job is to keep inviting it.

Chronic fatigue, fertility, emotional trauma, autoimmune responses

How the brain and body converge in complex patterns—and the hope of repatterning

When people think of chronic fatigue, fertility struggles, lingering emotional trauma, or autoimmune conditions, they often see them as separate problems requiring separate solutions. But modern neuroscience and psychoneuroimmunology reveal that these seemingly different issues often intersect within the same core system: the brain's regulation of stress, safety, and healing.

What connects them all is how the nervous system—especially under chronic or unresolved stress—recalibrates the entire body's priorities.

When the brain detects even subtle, ongoing threat (through past trauma patterns, high allostatic load, or subconscious hypervigilance), it shifts resources away from long-term repair, fertility, or robust energy production, and into protective short-term modes.

This is not psychological weakness—it is hardwired evolutionary biology.

But what was meant to be temporary can become chronic, leading to patterns where fatigue deepens, immune balance falters, reproductive cycles destabilize, and emotional triggers loop without full resolution.

Chronic fatigue: The energy shutdown response

Chronic fatigue is not only about mitochondrial inefficiency or low iron—it often emerges as the body's way of conserving resources in the face of perceived chronic threat.

Persistent sympathetic activation (fight or flight) eventually leads to parasympathetic "freeze" dominance, a state of shutdown meant to survive overwhelming situations by minimizing energy expenditure.

The brain begins down-regulating metabolism, muscle repair, and even neurotransmitter turnover to keep reserves in place for emergency needs.

Through neural repatterning, hypnosis, somatic retraining, and daily micro-signals of safety (like breathwork, rhythm, and gentle movement), the nervous system can be guided to interpret the environment as safe again, allowing it to lift energy-saving constraints and gradually restore robust vitality.

Fertility: Neuroendocrine permission vs. shutdown

Fertility challenges often highlight this same dynamic in another dimension.

Reproductive hormones like GnRH, LH, FSH, estrogen, and progesterone are tightly regulated by the hypothalamus—a part of the brain that is also a master detector of stress and safety cues.

Under chronic perceived threat, the hypothalamus may suppress reproductive signals because pregnancy is not a biologically wise choice when the system senses survival is under question.

This is why approaches that soothe the limbic system, balance the autonomic nervous system, and reduce subconscious hypervigilance (through targeted trance, emotional integration, and daily parasympathetic practices) often lead to improvements—even when purely medical interventions had stalled.

In many women, gentle neuroendocrine recalibration results in more regular cycles, improved ovulatory signals, and higher implantation potential. Similarly, men may see improvements in parameters tied to testosterone, sperm quality, and emotional steadiness, all intimately connected to chronic stress physiology.

Emotional trauma: The loop that feeds the body's alarm

Unresolved emotional trauma is not only a memory—it is a physiological imprint.

The amygdala and hippocampus encode emotional events with sensory richness, preparing the body to detect similar dangers in the future.

If these memories are never fully processed or "completed" (as often happens in overwhelming situations where fight/flight fails), the body carries forward micro-responses: muscular guarding, altered breath patterns, chronic low-grade inflammation.

These loops keep the nervous system primed, maintaining cortisol and adrenaline at subtle elevations, which then:

Suppress long-term cellular repair,

Disrupt digestion and nutrient absorption,

Contribute to energy shutdown,

And interfere with balanced immune surveillance.

Integrative trance work, targeted visualization, and somatic release techniques can help "finish" the story the body is still trying to protect against—allowing the nervous system to finally downshift into peace.

Autoimmune responses: When defense becomes misdirected

Autoimmunity is a striking example of the body's defenses becoming overly vigilant, attacking internal tissues as if they were foreign threats.

Research shows links between:

Early chronic stress or trauma and later autoimmune incidence,

Persistent low-level limbic alarm and altered cytokine profiles,

Gut barrier and microbiome shifts tied to sympathetic overdrive and stress hormones.

In practical terms, when the body never fully exits defensive mode, the immune system is more likely to misinterpret signals, fail to regulate inflammation, and continue patterns of inappropriate attack.

Protocols that retrain the brain-body relationship—through subconscious reprogramming, guided imagery of immune modulation, and daily lifestyle signals of calm—can often help reduce symptom flares, stabilize energy, and restore a more intelligent immune discernment.

A unified lens on healing

Though these conditions might appear disparate on a medical chart, they often share a common story:

The nervous system has learned (often for good reason in the past) that the world is not fully safe.

As a result, it conserves energy, suspends reproduction, heightens immune reactivity, and holds emotional residues close.

The power of combining trance therapy, visualization, lifestyle alignment, frequency support, and gentle somatic integration lies in teaching the brain a new possibility:

"It is safe now. You can heal. You can rebalance. You can create again—whether that means more energy, a new life, or simply a calm heart."

Healing is rarely about forcing the body to comply. It is about inviting the nervous system to see that it no longer needs to protect so fiercely—And watching how energy, fertility, emotional lightness, and immune clarity naturally return.

Insights from years of regenerative medicine and hypnosis practice

What the science and thousands of patient journeys have revealed

After decades in regenerative medicine, cellular health, and clinical hypnosis, one truth stands above all else:

The human body is inherently designed to heal, adapt, and regenerate—if we can create the right internal conditions.

Most people think of regeneration in purely physical terms: wound healing, tissue repair, immune recalibration. But as years of working with patients have shown, true regeneration often begins at a far deeper level—inside the nervous system, the subconscious mind, and the subtle patterns that determine whether the body stays in protection or shifts into growth.

Whether someone came to see me for hormone imbalance, lingering injury, autoimmune activity, trauma after grief, or simply unexplained exhaustion, the same principle applied:

If the brain remained on alert—due to old emotional residues, hidden beliefs of unworthiness, or a body that still expected harm—the physiology could not fully prioritize repair.

But once we gently guided the subconscious into safety, reframed the meaning of long-held patterns, and reinforced this with daily signals of calm and coherence, the body almost always began to find its own way back.

Years of practice have also taught me this:

It is never too late.

The nervous system can change, even after decades of rigidity.

Older adults often experience some of the most dramatic shifts, because their bodies have long been waiting for permission to move out of defense.

5 remarkable cases of profound regeneration and trauma resolution using HypnoCell®

Each of these stories highlights patients in their 60s to 70s, people who often believed (or were told) they were simply "too old to expect much change." Yet under a carefully structured program blending lifestyle shifts, daily frequency support, and deep subconscious recalibration through the HypnoCell® process, their bodies and minds surprised them.

Case 1: Recovering from a decade of chronic pain and lost mobility

Patient: Elena, 68, retired school administrator.

Background: Had lived with chronic hip and lower back pain since her mid-50s after a minor car accident. Despite normal scans, she walked with guarded stiffness, needed daily painkillers, and believed her "age just meant living with it."

Approach:

Used gentle hypnotic regression to trace the original somatic holding—not just the accident, but a lifetime pattern of "bracing against criticism."

Paired this with vibrational sound bowl sessions at home and daily slow walking with breath synchronization.

Outcome:

Within 2 months, began spontaneously moving more freely.

By 5 months, had reduced her pain medication by 75% and was gardening again.

Told her daughter: "I feel like the tension finally melted off my bones."

Case 2: Emotional grief transformed, thyroid function stabilized

Patient: Jorge, 72, widowed, living with Hashimoto's for over 20 years.

Background: Labs had long been stable on medication, but he suffered persistent fatigue, mild tremors, and a sense of emotional flatness since losing his wife.

Approach:

Integrated HypnoCell® subconscious work focusing on gently "inviting back joy," coupled with daily sessions using healing frequency tracks designed for endocrine support.

Practiced simple heart-focused breathing with visualization of light expanding in his chest.

Outcome:

By month 4, reported brighter moods, less internal trembling, and returned to playing guitar.

His endocrinologist noted slightly more stable antibody markers for the first time in years.

Most movingly, he said: "I don't just exist anymore. I catch myself smiling at the sunrise."

Case 3: Long-standing trauma resolved, digestion restored

Patient: Nuria, 63, former business owner, long history of IBS and acid reflux, plus insomnia tied to childhood emotional trauma.

Background: Had spent decades believing her gut issues were simply structural or hereditary. Sleep was shallow and fragmented for over 20 years.

Approach:

Used HypnoCell® sessions to explore her gut's "role" as a subconscious vessel for unspoken fears.

Introduced daily vibration bowl use over the abdomen, plus self-hypnosis scripts visualizing her digestive tract as calm, pink, and fluid.

Outcome:

Within weeks, she noticed sleeping 90 minutes longer each night without waking.

By month 6, experienced fewer urgent gut episodes and even tolerated foods she'd avoided for decades.

Said with tears: "I didn't know it was possible to live without always clutching my stomach."

Case 4: Rheumatoid arthritis flares diminished and emotional openness returned

Patient: Daniel, 70, former mechanical engineer, living with Rheumatoid Arthritis (RA) for over 15 years.

Background: Managed on biologics but still had frequent flares and had become emotionally shut down, avoiding gatherings because he felt "irritable with people."

Approach:

HypnoCell® protocols focused on reframing subconscious narratives of self-punishment and "over-responsibility."

Layered with low-frequency sound therapy designed to help calm joint and tissue inflammation, practiced alongside gentle parasympathetic breathing.

Outcome:

By month 3, noted milder, shorter flares even with reduced medication.

Began attending weekly lunches with old friends again, saying:"It's not just my joints — my heart feels less locked up."

Case 5: A journey from cognitive fog and shame to clarity and self-compassion

Patient: Beatriz, 66, a retired librarian.

Background: Came in worried about memory slips and what she called "slowness," haunted by family history of dementia. Also carried deep shame over past mistakes, feeding a loop of stress and forgetfulness.

Approach:

Worked through HypnoCell® sessions that safely accessed subconscious memories tied to long-standing guilt, gently rewriting internal narratives of worth.

Added a daily ritual with healing frequencies and a personal anchor — placing her hand on her head and saying softly, "My mind is safe. My mind is growing."

Outcome:

Within 4 months, described sharper recall and more confidence in social conversations.

Felt more emotionally regulated, telling her daughter:"I still have little lapses, but I no longer panic. It's like my brain and heart are on the same team again."

The deeper insight

These cases illustrate the profound adaptability that still lives in the brain and body — even decades into life.They reveal that while structural changes may come with age, the nervous system's capacity to reorganize around new patterns, to release protective contractions, and to prioritize restoration is incredibly resilient.

What allowed these shifts was not brute force, but a multi-layered approach:

Creating consistent signals of safety and possibility through breath, lifestyle, visualization, sound, and daily anchors.

Accessing subconscious programming gently and precisely, helping the brain learn it no longer needed to guard so fiercely.

Inviting tissues, immune functions, and even hormones to recalibrate under this new internal climate.

The most hopeful truth from all these years of work?

No matter how long someone has lived in patterns of pain, exhaustion, or quiet suffering, the brain and body still recognize the language of safety, still respond to permission to heal —and often surprise us with just how far they can come back.

Chapter 10

Building your neural regeneration plan

One of the greatest breakthroughs in modern neuroscience is the understanding that the brain is plastic, adaptable, and always capable of remodeling itself. This process—called neuroplasticity—means your nervous system is constantly reshaping its circuits, reassigning resources, and adjusting how it communicates with the immune, endocrine, and even digestive systems.

What many people don't realize is that neuroplasticity is not automatically positive. Chronic stress, persistent negative focus, unresolved trauma, and lifestyle habits that reinforce vigilance can wire your brain more deeply into defense, exhaustion, or inflammation.

The goal of a neural regeneration plan is to flip this pattern—to deliberately create an inner environment that favors safety, coherence, and cellular repair. In other words, you are training your brain to prioritize healing over survival mode.

This isn't something that happens from one hypnosis session, meditation, or supplement. It's a systematic approach, aligning subconscious reprogramming with daily signals that continually tell your nervous system:

"It is safe now. You can rebalance. You can restore."

The core components of a neural regeneration plan

Your personalized plan weaves together four critical layers:

1. Targeted neural rewiring (subconscious work)

This involves:

Self-hypnosis or guided hypnosis sessions that access the subconscious, where long-standing emotional, behavioral, or protective patterns are stored.

Visualization techniques that install new templates of calm, repair, or immune balance—training your brain's predictive coding to expect a different outcome.

Somatic cues (like gentle hand placement or slow rocking) layered into these sessions to integrate body memory.

Why it matters:

The subconscious governs around 90-95% of your autonomic and behavioral patterns. If this layer still perceives danger, no amount of conscious intention can fully override it.

2. Daily lifestyle inputs as neural messages

Lifestyle is not background. It is continuous programming for your nervous system.

Nutrition that reduces neuroinflammation and stabilizes blood sugar, preventing spikes that feed anxiety circuits.

Regular movement to stimulate BDNF (brain-derived neurotrophic factor), enhancing synaptic growth and flexibility.

Consistent sleep that allows your brain's glymphatic system to clear out metabolic waste, consolidate new neural pathways, and regulate emotional centers.

Why it matters:

Every meal, every bout of movement, every sleep cycle either strengthens circuits of calm and repair—or reinforces vigilance and chronic shutdown.

3. Breath, frequency, and subtle vibration

Supporting the brain through:

Breathwork that intentionally slows and lengthens exhales, activating the vagus nerve and parasympathetic system.

Gentle vibrational therapies (like sound bowls, binaural beats, or frequency tracks) that entrain your brain into slower waves (alpha, theta, delta) where neuroplastic change and cellular restoration thrive.

Why it matters:

You are literally using sound and breath as biological tuning forks, shifting your entire internal state from hyper-alert to receptive and regenerative.

4. Micro-emotional and social safety practices

Because the brain is wired to heal only when it feels safe:

Using brief daily scripts or anchors ("I am safe now. My body knows how to repair.") paired with calming touch or gentle rocking.

Spending time in environments that reduce threat cues—nature, warm lighting, kind company.

Actively practicing moments of savoring small pleasures, teaching your limbic system to lean toward positivity.

Why it matters:

Repetition of tiny moments of safety re-patterns the amygdala and hippocampus, shrinking emotional overreaction and building resilience.

How to start: Mapping your own plan

Identify one core area you want to shift (fatigue, inflammation, pain, emotional hyper-reactivity, etc).

Choose two small daily rituals—like a short visualization plus a breath anchor before bed.

Schedule deeper sessions weekly, whether that's self-hypnosis, a sound bath, or guided trance therapy.

Journal simple observations, reinforcing new narratives (e.g., "My body felt lighter today. I moved without bracing.")

This is not a rigid protocol. It's about creating a reliable rhythm of safety, meaning, and repair signals that your nervous system can trust and start to internalize.

Remember: Regeneration is a Biological Tendency

Your brain and body want to heal.

Neurons want to find more efficient connections.

Immune cells want to balance instead of overreact.

Hormones want to return to circadian harmony.

A neural regeneration plan is simply the structure that gives them permission and repetition—until repair becomes the new baseline.

This is your roadmap to transform neuroplasticity from something that accidentally maintains stress...into something that actively builds calm, clarity, and resilience.

One small, consistent cue at a time.

Customizing your own neuroplastic healing roadmap

Designing a personal path to rewire, restore, and renew

Healing is never truly one-size-fits-all. While the principles of neuroplasticity, mind-body recalibration, and subconscious repatterning apply to everyone, the details of how you activate these processes must fit your life, your patterns, and your unique biology.

This is why it's so powerful to build a personalized neuroplastic healing roadmap—a clear, flexible structure that guides your brain and body from patterns of vigilance or stagnation toward safety, growth, and deep repair.

Think of it as drawing your own set of daily and weekly instructions for your nervous system—teaching it, over and over, that it is safe to downshift from protection into regeneration.

Why "customization" is essential for true change

The brain does not heal through abstract concepts. It responds to what feels real, believable, and consistently reinforced. That's why it's crucial your roadmap is:

Aligned with your personal life rhythms.

If you work long shifts or have young children, your plan might center on micro-practices throughout the day, rather than long uninterrupted sessions.

Matched to your nervous system's current capacity.

For some, starting with gentle breath anchoring feels right; for others, immersive guided hypnosis is welcomed. There's no single starting point.

Rooted in what emotionally resonates with you.

If you find nature deeply soothing, walks or grounding might anchor your plan. If music shifts your state quickly, frequency work becomes your primary tool.

This is how you make your plan sustainable—and how your subconscious begins to trust the process enough to allow real rewiring.

Elements of your personal roadmap

Here are core components most effective neuroplastic plans weave together. As you customize yours, think about which areas feel most relevant or accessible for you right now.

1. **Daily regulation practices**

Small, repeatable actions that cue your nervous system to settle.

Examples:

4-7-8 or box breathing patterns twice daily

Short somatic scans (checking and softening your jaw, shoulders, belly)

A 5-minute gentle stretching or swaying ritual before bed

2. **Focused subconscious work**

At least several times a week, carve out intentional time to address deep patterns.

Examples:

Self-hypnosis using personalized scripts tied to your specific symptom or goal

Regenerative meditation that combines visualization with slow breathing

Using frequency tracks designed to sustain theta/delta states for subconscious access

3. **Neuro-nourishment & physical support**

Because your brain can't rewire effectively if starved of resources.

Examples:

Ensuring healthy fats (omega-3s), colorful antioxidants, magnesium-rich greens

Prioritizing consistent sleep windows to consolidate neural changes

Gentle morning movement to stimulate BDNF and signal metabolic readiness

4. **Emotional & social safety**

Chronic threat patterns often begin or persist in isolation or emotional suppression.

Examples:

Texting or calling someone you trust each day

Keeping a short "gratitude / today's small joys" list

Giving yourself 5 minutes nightly to place a hand on your chest and simply breathe, telling your system: "I am here, safe with myself."

5. Anchors & triggers for rapid reset

Physical cues you use anytime stress spikes—tying a specific small action to your new calm state.

Examples:

Pressing thumb and forefinger together while slowly exhaling

Lightly tapping your heart center three times while repeating, "It's okay to release."

Humming softly to stimulate the vagus nerve and reduce limbic alarm.

How to Start Building Your Custom Plan

Choose one core outcome you'd like to address first (better sleep, calmer digestion, less emotional reactivity, more energy).

Pick 2–3 simple daily signals that cue your nervous system toward safety.

Schedule at least one deeper session each week for guided or self-hypnosis, vibrational therapy, or immersive visualization.

Stack habits together. For example, listen to a calming frequency track while doing your breathwork at night.

Reassess every few weeks: notice small changes in how you feel or react. Adjust or add practices as needed.

Remember: Flexibility is built in

Your roadmap is not a rigid set of demands. It is a living, evolving guide, adapting as your nervous system becomes more stable and receptive.

Some weeks, your brain might be ready for deep subconscious sessions.

Other times, simply maintaining breath anchors and gentle self-talk might be enough.

Over time, you may expand from regulating single symptoms to rewriting larger emotional or identity patterns.

This adaptability is what makes your plan powerful—and sustainable enough to become a lifelong foundation for resilience and renewal.

A personalized neuroplastic roadmap is like drawing a new set of neural pathways—One tiny, repeated step at a time, until your brain and body know the way by heart.

Tracking results and supporting change

How to measure progress and reinforce your brain's new pathways

One of the most overlooked—but crucial—steps in any neuroplastic healing journey is the simple act of tracking and observing your progress.

Why? Because the nervous system is programmed to pay attention to what feels threatening, negative, or familiar. If you don't intentionally notice small shifts—less pain, a calmer stomach, lighter moods—your brain is likely to default back to scanning for problems.

Documenting your results, no matter how subtle, sends a powerful subconscious signal:

"Change is happening. Healing is underway. This new pattern is real."

It's also essential for another reason: by recording improvements and insights, you reinforce the new neural pathways you're building, making them more dominant and automatic over time.

Why tracking is a neuroplastic tool, not just a diary

Each time you notice a new ease in your body, a reduction in symptoms, or a moment of emotional steadiness, you're helping your brain encode the experience as meaningful.

Repeatedly registering these positives strengthens synapses tied to calm, safety, and optimism—literally wiring them into your neural architecture.

Tracking also reduces the common phenomenon of "healing amnesia," where people forget how far they've come because the brain adapts quickly to improvements and resumes looking for threats.

How to track: Gentle, sustainable methods

This doesn't have to be a burdensome chore. It's about brief, consistent noticing.

1. **The daily two-line check**

Each evening, jot down:

One small shift or improvement you noticed (even if it's simply, "Felt more hopeful this morning.")

One area you want to keep supporting (e.g., "Still tension in my neck under stress.")

This trains your mind to balance awareness of progress with gentle focus on continued goals.

2. Weekly quick-reflection

Once a week, spend 5 minutes noting:

What feels better or easier?

What still needs support?

Any surprising emotional or lifestyle changes?

Over time, these notes become a powerful record of transformation—reminding you, during tough days, that your body and brain are changing.

3. Using a symptom / ease scale

Many people find it helpful to pick a simple 1-10 scale for key markers like:

Fatigue

Digestive flares

Pain levels

Anxiety surges

Rate them every few days, but equally note positive states, like:

Calm (0–10)

Energy on waking (0–10)

Ease of social interactions (0–10)

This avoids the trap of only watching for problems.

Supporting change: Reinforcement techniques

Tracking is about more than measurement. It also actively supports the brain in consolidating new patterns. Here's how to build that reinforcement:

Celebrate micro-shifts

Even tiny wins matter. If you had one day of less pain, one meal without bloating, or one interaction that felt more relaxed—acknowledge it.

Say to yourself:

"That's new. That's evidence of change."

Each small recognition acts like a dopamine spark that makes the brain more eager to repeat the new pattern.

Pair with anchors

When you track a positive, reinforce it somatically. Place a hand on your heart, breathe slowly, or lightly squeeze thumb to forefinger. This ties the new perception to a physical anchor, deepening the subconscious imprint.

Keep a healing highlights page

Start a page in your journal simply titled "Signs of Healing." Each week, add anything big or small.

"More calm at dinner with family."

"Fell asleep faster three nights."

"Woke up with less jaw tension."

On harder days, read this page. It trains your brain to see the trajectory, not just momentary dips.

Why this matters for long-term rewiring

Neuroplastic change requires evidence and repetition.When your subconscious sees patterns of improvement written down, revisited, and celebrated, it accepts:

"This is the new normal. I can stabilize here."

Without this intentional noticing, the brain often slips back into its old vigilance pathways—simply because those circuits were used more often in the past.

Healing is a journey of millions of micro-signals.Tracking them—gently, without judgment—turns them into a clear, compelling story your nervous system can trust.

When to seek professional guidance

Why healing deep patterns often needs expert navigation—and how this can transform your progress

While daily self-hypnosis, visualization, breathwork, and frequency practices are incredibly powerful tools, there are times when working with a trained professional is not just helpful—it's the wisest, fastest, and often the only way to reach the levels of change your body and subconscious truly need.

Many people begin their journey using self-guided methods, only to find they reach a plateau. Symptoms may lessen but never fully resolve, or old emotional loops keep resurfacing under stress. This isn't because they've failed—it's because the deepest, most entrenched patterns usually live in areas of the mind that we can't fully reach or restructure on our own.

Why the most profound shifts often require professional help

Here's what I've seen repeatedly across years of practice in regenerative medicine and clinical hypnosis—and what neuroscience clearly explains:

Your subconscious protections are sophisticated. They were formed to keep you safe, often decades ago. They know how to hide, redirect, or even rationalize themselves to keep from being dismantled. A skilled practitioner can spot these protective strategies—like sudden mental fog, subtle muscle tensing, or deflection—and gently guide you through them.

Deep trance states are more easily achieved with a professional. While self-hypnosis and guided recordings can take you into moderate depths (alpha, light theta), the very patterns you need to rewrite often live deeper—in subconscious levels that require skilled pacing, advanced metaphor work, or specific neural pattern interrupts to safely access.

Complex emotional material is hard to hold alone. When unresolved trauma, grief, or shame surfaces, it's easy to either flood (becoming overwhelmed) or shut down (numbing out). A professional creates a secure container, reads your subtle signals, and knows precisely how to titrate the process so your nervous system stays safe, integrated, and capable of true reprocessing.

A trained hypnotherapist or mind-body professional can customize the approach uniquely to your history, body responses, and subconscious language.

They see connections and unconscious metaphors you may never realize are driving your symptoms—helping target root patterns far more precisely than general scripts.

When should you consider professional guidance?

If you notice:

You've hit a plateau after weeks or months of trying on your own—symptoms won't budge further or keep cycling back.

You experience strong emotional flooding (like panic, deep sadness, or old traumatic sensations) when doing self-hypnosis or meditation.

You have long-standing or complex issues like autoimmune patterns, chronic pain with no clear injury, or trauma stored in the body (e.g., sudden tears, digestive disruptions, or muscle tightening without obvious reason).

You feel a persistent sense of "I'm stuck, I can't do this alone."

Or if you simply want:

Faster, more elegant results—someone guiding you past your mind's defenses and directly into deep subconscious recalibration.

Tailored metaphors, imagery, and layered suggestions that specifically fit your personal history and physiology.

The relief of having someone hold the process for you, so your nervous system doesn't have to navigate and heal at the same time.

Why it's not a sign of failure—but profound self-compassion

Seeking professional guidance isn't giving up your power. It's actually one of the most courageous, intelligent acts of self-care you can take.

Because deep patterns of vigilance, fatigue, reproductive shutdown, immune hyperactivity, or emotional guarding weren't created alone—they were built in complex life contexts, often when you had limited support.

Letting an experienced practitioner guide you is how you give your nervous system something it may never have had:

A safe, expertly held space to fully unravel old patterns, to rewire without fear of overwhelm, and to discover new ways of being that you can't always find by yourself.

Your subconscious mind knows how to heal—but sometimes it needs a skilled hand to unlock the door, hold the light, and keep it steady while your deepest systems learn a new way to live.

The future of regenerative hypnotherapy

Reimagining healing through the brain's Remarkable power to restore

We stand at a remarkable crossroads in medicine, neuroscience, and human potential. For decades, healthcare was largely divided: the mind was treated separately from the body, emotions were often sidelined, and the brain was wrongly assumed to be mostly fixed after childhood.

Now, thanks to decades of neuroplasticity research, psychoneuroimmunology breakthroughs, and the integration of subtle energetic models, we know this simply isn't true.

The brain remains adaptable for life.

The subconscious can be re-educated.

The nervous system can learn to interpret the world differently, trading chronic defense for cellular repair.

Where regenerative hypnotherapy is heading

Regenerative hypnotherapy is not simply about reducing stress or managing symptoms. It is rapidly evolving into a precise therapeutic technology, one that:

Targets the deep root drivers of chronic patterns—emotional, neurological, even immune-related—through direct subconscious and autonomic recalibration.

Uses advanced tools like brainwave frequency entrainment, subtle vibration, personalized metaphor work, and cutting-edge knowledge of predictive brain coding to restructure how the body allocates resources toward healing.

Complements (and in some cases amplifies) physical regenerative therapies—whether stem cell approaches, peptide protocols, or lifestyle-based cellular optimization—by ensuring the nervous system is not sabotaging them with hidden threat responses.

A future of integration and empowerment

Imagine a future where:

A patient recovering from autoimmune flares doesn't just take immune-modulating drugs, but also undergoes tailored hypnotherapy sessions to teach their subconscious that it no longer needs to launch overreactions.

Women struggling with unexplained fertility challenges use personalized subconscious rewiring sessions to restore neuroendocrine signals that once suppressed ovulation out of perceived stress.

Older adults once resigned to "slowing down" harness structured hypnotic and frequency programs to sharpen cognition, rebuild resilience, and literally remodel synaptic pathways for clarity and calm.

This is not speculative hope—it is already happening.Studies and thousands of patient experiences show us that when the subconscious receives new instructions, when the limbic system finally believes "it is safe," the entire body shifts:

Inflammation reduces.

Digestion normalizes.

Hormones rebalance.

Sleep deepens.

Cellular repair genes upregulate.

And perhaps most importantly: the person feels new. Not simply less symptomatic, but more alive, emotionally open, and connected to their body's innate intelligence.

Your invitation to be part of this new paradigm

The future of regenerative hypnotherapy is here for anyone ready to step beyond passive hope and become an active participant in their own restoration.

Whether through working with a skilled practitioner who can expertly navigate your subconscious architecture, or by using daily tools and frequency support to reinforce your new patterns, you hold extraordinary influence over how your mind and body heal.

The deepest message of this entire approach is simple yet revolutionary:

Your brain is not broken.

Your body is not stuck.

They are waiting for the right signals—delivered with care, repetition, and meaning—to show you how powerfully they can regenerate.

· · • · • • • • · ·

Appendix 1
Sample brainwave frequency charts

Understanding brainwaves is like learning the language of your brain's internal rhythms. Each pattern of electrical activity reflects a different state of consciousness, each with its own profound effects on your body, your mind, and your capacity to regenerate.

Modern neurofeedback, EEG studies, and countless hypnosis and meditation trials show that specific brainwave states correlate with unique capacities for repair, learning, and emotional integration.

By knowing these patterns—and intentionally guiding yourself into them through breath, sound, hypnosis, or frequency work—you're essentially becoming an architect of your own neuroplastic landscape.

Why These Frequencies Matter for Regeneration

Delta

When your brain is in delta, it's prioritizing body-level repair: clearing metabolic waste, optimizing growth hormone and immune balance, repairing tissues. Deep sleep and certain deep hypnosis states promote this. Without enough delta dominance, physical healing is compromised.

Theta

Theta is the gateway to the subconscious. It's where your brain becomes most receptive to new patterns—whether that's releasing stored trauma, accepting new beliefs about safety, or creatively solving problems beyond the reach of ordinary logic. This is why so many hypnosis protocols, including aspects of HypnoCell®, target this range.

Alpha

Alpha acts like a bridge between conscious and subconscious, allowing calm receptivity. In alpha, stress chemistry lowers, and your brain integrates emotions and ideas more fluidly. Many regenerative meditation practices aim to hover here.

Beta

Beta is necessary—it's how you navigate work, conversations, planning. But excessive beta, especially high beta (20–30 Hz), is tied to vigilance, chronic worry, shallow breath, and reduced capacity for deeper healing processes. That's why consciously dropping into alpha-theta states is so critical for those with chronic conditions.

Brainwave	Frequency Range	Typical State	Healing Relevance
Delta (δ)	0.5 – 4 Hz	Deep, dreamless sleep, subconscious bodily repair	Cellular regeneration, immune recalibration, deep tissue healing, hormonal reset
Theta (θ)	4 – 8 Hz	Light sleep, deep meditation, trance, vivid imagery	Optimal for subconscious reprogramming, emotional memory processing, creativity
Alpha (α)	8 – 12 Hz	Relaxed alertness, calm focus, wakeful rest	Stress reduction, integrative processing, opening pathways for learning
Beta (β)	12 – 30 Hz	Normal waking state, problem-solving, active thinking	Necessary for daily function, but sustained high beta correlates with anxiety, vigilance
Gamma (γ)	30 – 100 Hz	High-level information integration, moments of insight	Tied to peak states and synchrony across brain regions (less central for subconscious healing work, but valuable for cognitive integration)

How this informs your practice

When you look at these frequencies, it becomes clear why:

Binaural beats or isochronic tones tuned to theta encourage subconscious openness.

Gentle vibration bowls can drop you from beta into alpha within minutes.

Slow breathing lengthens your alpha states, making it easier to shift into theta.

Sleep hygiene (dark, cool environments, consistent bedtimes) protects your delta time, giving your body the nightly restoration it craves.

· · ● · ● · · ● · · · ·

Appendix 2
Glossary of key terms

This glossary gives you concise, plain-language definitions of important concepts used throughout this book. It's designed so you can revisit it anytime to refresh your understanding—because many of these ideas are new to people, and their power lies in truly grasping how they work.

Neuroplasticity

The brain's lifelong ability to change its structure and function in response to experience, thought patterns, emotions, learning, or injury. Neuroplasticity is why new habits can eventually overwrite old ones, and why subconscious healing methods can lead to lasting biological shifts.

Psychoneuroimmunology (PNI)

A scientific field exploring how thoughts and emotions influence the nervous system, immune function, and endocrine (hormonal) responses. It shows that stress, belief, and emotional states can directly affect inflammation, healing speed, and even genetic expression.

Subconscious Mind

The part of your mind operating below conscious awareness, managing habits, emotions, protective patterns, and much of your body's automatic functions. Hypnosis and visualization work by communicating directly with this level to install new instructions.

Hypnosis (Clinical Hypnosis)

A therapeutic technique that guides the mind into a focused, highly receptive state (often linked to alpha and theta brainwaves), where it is easier to update subconscious patterns, reduce protective reflexes, and plant suggestions that favor healing.

Self-Hypnosis

A method of intentionally guiding yourself into a mild trance state to deliver positive suggestions, rehearse healing imagery, or calm overactive neural loops. It builds on the same principles as guided hypnosis but is done independently.

Frequency Entrainment

Using sound patterns (like binaural beats, isochronic tones, or vibration bowls) to align brainwave activity to a desired frequency, such as theta for subconscious processing or delta for cellular repair. It "nudges" the brain into specific states.

Vagus Nerve

The longest cranial nerve, running from the brainstem through the heart, lungs, and gut. It's a primary conduit for the parasympathetic nervous system (rest-and-repair). Stimulating the vagus nerve through slow breath, humming, or gentle vibration increases calm and supports regeneration.

Allostatic Load

The wear and tear on the body from chronic stress, including hormonal shifts, immune dysregulation, and neural patterns that maintain vigilance even after danger has passed.

Neuroendocrine Axis

The complex communication network between the brain (especially the hypothalamus), the pituitary gland, and peripheral glands (like thyroid, adrenals, ovaries or testes). Stress, safety, and subconscious beliefs directly influence this axis, affecting hormones, metabolism, and fertility.

Limbic System

A set of brain structures (including the amygdala and hippocampus) that process emotion, memory, and perceived threat. Overactive limbic circuits often underlie chronic anxiety, digestive issues, and autoimmune patterns.

Regeneration

The biological process of repairing or replacing damaged cells and tissues. In this book's context, it refers to creating the neural, emotional, and cellular conditions that favor true restoration over ongoing protection or degeneration.

HypnoCell®

A specialized method that combines clinical hypnosis, principles of neuroplasticity, psychoneuroimmunology, and regenerative lifestyle strategies to trace symptoms back to their root informational signals, then reframe and install new instructions for healing at subconscious and cellular levels.

Anchor Technique

A physical or sensory cue (like touching your heart, pressing fingers together, or humming) intentionally paired with a calm or healing state, so later doing the action automatically triggers that state by association. A core tool in neuroplastic self-regulation.

Heart Rate Variability (HRV)

A measure of variation in time between heartbeats. Greater HRV generally indicates better adaptability and resilience, showing your nervous system can shift smoothly between states of alertness and rest.

Visualization

Using the mind's eye to imagine specific scenes, sensations, or bodily processes. The brain often reacts to vivid imagery as if it's real, activating circuits tied to calm, immune function, or tissue healing.

Tip:Come back to this glossary anytime you need to refresh a concept—these aren't just definitions, they're the foundational keys to understanding how your brain and body can truly regenerate.

About the author

Dr. Lucy Coleman is a medical doctor specialized in high-complexity fertility and human reproduction, with extensive expertise in guiding patients through some of the most intricate dimensions of health and healing. Over the past 14 years, she has developed and refined the **HypnoCell® system**—a pioneering approach that combines therapeutic hypnosis with cellular regeneration, designed to help patients move beyond chronic illness and into lasting restoration.

Dr. Coleman's passion for integrating the science of medicine with the deeper potentials of the mind has led her to advanced training with leaders in the field. She has studied under **Dr. Brian Weiss**, internationally recognized for his work on the mind-body connection; practiced yoga-based therapeutic principles with **Doug Hayward**, master teacher of embodied healing; and expanded her expertise in subconscious reprogramming at the **Path Institute in Houston** under **Doyle Ward**.

Her clinical experience, paired with her personal dedication to continuous study, has allowed her to create programs that go beyond standard symptom management—offering patients pathways to rewire long-held protective patterns, rebalance immune and endocrine functions, and cultivate profound neuroplastic change.

Dr. Coleman now shares this evolving work worldwide through the HypnoCell® platform, workshops, and online programs, helping people unlock their innate capacity to regenerate on every level: neurological, cellular, and emotional.

She continues to live her philosophy daily—combining a scientific lens with deep respect for the body's intelligence and a belief that true healing always begins from within.

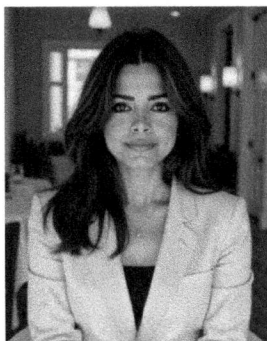

Thank you for taking the time to explore this book—a work crafted with care, drawing on the most innovative, evidence-based insights in neuroplasticity, psychoneuroimmunology, and subconscious healing. It is my hope that these pages have opened a door to new possibilities for your body, your mind, and your future.

If you'd like to continue this journey, discover more about the HypnoCell® approach, or access additional tools and resources, I warmly invite you to visit hypnocell.com. There you'll find guidance, specialized programs, and the latest updates designed to help you activate your own innate capacity for regeneration.

Thank you again for reading, for your openness, and for daring to believe in your body's extraordinary ability to heal.

May this be the beginning of a new chapter—one grounded in science, possibility, and profound self-renewal.

www.ingramcontent.com/pod-product-compliance
Lightning Source LLC
Chambersburg PA
CBHW070802290326
41931CB00011BA/2107